ESSENTIALS OF BIOINFORMATICS: AN INTRODUCTION FOR UNDERGRADUATES

ESSENTIALS OF BIOINFORMATICS: AN INTRODUCTION FOR UNDERGRADUATES

Edited by

Dr. Akansha Singh

Delve
PUBLISHING

www.delvepublishing.com

Essentials of Bioinformatics: An Introduction for Undergraduates

Dr. Akansha Singh

Delve Publishing
224 Shoreacres Road
Burlington, ON L7L 2H2
Canada
www.delvepublishing.com
Email: orders@arclereducation.com

ISBN: 978-1-77469-801-3 (Hardcover)

ABOUT THE EDITOR

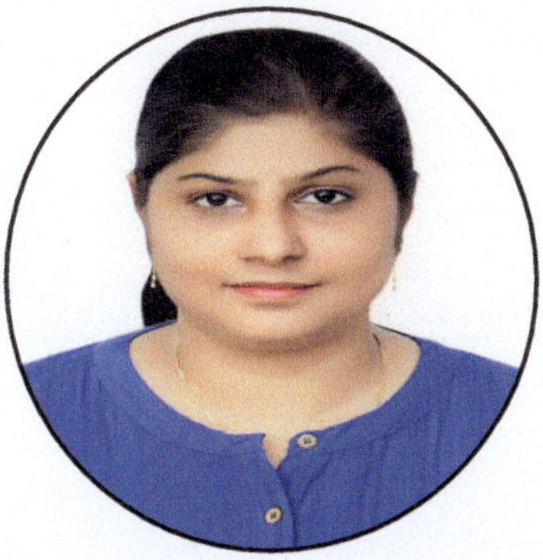

Dr. Akansha Singh is presently working as Project Scientist in Department of Genetics and Plant Breeding, Institute of Agricultural Sciences, Banaras Hindu University, India. She has also worked as Postdoctoral fellow, Mumbai University and as Associate Professor, Department of Genetics and Plant Breeding, College of Agriculture, Parul University, India She has obtained her Ph.D. (Ag) in Genetics and Plant breeding from Banaras Hindu University in the year 2012. She has been Awarded with ICAR, senior research fellowship in 2010 to pursue PhD. She has authored numerous national and international publications in journals of repute.

TABLE OF CONTENTS

LIST OF FIGURES

ABSTRACT

For the last few decades, the incorporation of genetics, genomics, proteomics, and statistics into the field of bioinformatics has had a significant impact on both the field of biology and the field of medicine. Its primary application is in assisting with the modeling, forecasting, and analysis of enormous amounts of multidimensional biological data utilizing the most recent and cutting-edge computational technologies. Most life science students and researchers do not have the skills necessary to make effective use of this sophisticated technology, which is why bioinformatics is not yet widely incorporated in academic courses despite the fact that it holds enormous promise. This book was written after realizing a void in the market for a resource that could provide students and researchers with prior knowledge of biosciences to begin their studies. This book teaches students how to apply cutting-edge open-source tools to real-world biological problems, in contrast to the majority of bioinformatics textbooks, which focus primarily on theory. As a quick reference, you can make use of the included flowcharts and diagrams. As a result of this, the book is an excellent resource that students and young professionals can use in their pursuit of knowledge on this ever-changing topic.

PREFACE

In comparison to more established branches of biology, bioinformatics is a recent development. Bioinformatics has rapidly become an essential scientific field thanks to recent developments in chemistry, biology, engineering, sequencing, and state-of-the-art computer tools. Due to the exponential accumulation of sequencing data produced by numerous living species and soon more, accessing and analyzing tremendously complicated genomic information has become one of the most critical study challenges in current molecular biology and genetics. However, mining this huge genetic data, the size of which typically ranges from gigabytes to terabytes and is generated by whole genome, exome, or RNA sequencing, requires cutting-edge computing approaches. To address the enormous challenges of next-generation genomics, the development of multi-bioinformatics software requires the participation of not just biologists and statisticians, but also computer scientists.

Over the past couple of decades, several educational institutions have made state-of-the-art bioinformatics software freely available to the general public. Normal bench scientists have a hard time keeping up with the discipline since no single textbook covers all the bioinformatics tools and resources. The new textbook makes accessible a wide range of cutting-edge bioinformatics resources that may be used in this pivotal study.

This book is meant to serve as an introduction to the discipline of bioinformatics, guiding the reader through its fundamentals and exposing them to the many databases and software programs used to analyze biological systems ranging from genes to proteins. The theoretical foundations and practical uses of these strategies are discussed in length. In addition, it employs visual aids like charts and pictures to teach the readers how to increase their efficiency. The writers give comprehensive, precise, and step-by-step directions for a few frequent scenarios as examples of how to deal with a specific problem in the actual world. This book does not include step-by-step instructions on how to use any of the programs it discusses; instead, it delves into the history, intended use, and actual application of each one. Most of the computational methods discussed here may be accessed without cost or any preparation from the reader.

CHAPTER 1

ELEMENTS OF BIOLOGY

CONTENTS

1.1 INTRODUCTION

A large fraction of naturally occurring chemical components of the Earth is required for life. Hydrogen, carbon, nitrogen, and oxygen make up 99% of protoplasmic mass. Phosphorus and sulfur are essential components of nucleic acids and amino acids. Chlorine, potassium, magnesium, calcium, and phosphorus have fast ionization and influence membrane activity and osmotic potential. Metals play a function in protein structure in living beings. Hemoglobin needs iron, while chlorophyll needs magnesium. Prokaryotes need certain components. Methanogens require lanthanide rare earth (Kellis, 2014).

Most elements have only been directly biologically investigated in connection to their importance to human health, including a study on chickens, rats, and agriculturally significant plants. There is evidence that certain elements are essential to groups other than humans. However, little effort has been made to systematically study these groups to determine the effects of deficiency of uncommon elements. Knowledge for these groups is largely limited to information gathered incidentally while studying other aspects of each organism.

The noble gases helium, neon, argon, krypton, and xenon are nonreactive and have no known direct biological importance – albeit xenon, despite being considered "chemically neutral," has both anesthetic and neuroprotective side effects and can activate at least one human transcription factor. (Radon is radioactive). Some elements are exceedingly scarce on Earth surface; thus, any lifeform that relied on them would have a restricted habitat and maybe a short lifetime. Example: rhodium with tantalum. Some elements frequently substitute for other, more common elements in molecular structures, such as bromine for chlorine or tungsten for molybdenum. Occasionally, this exchange has no biological impact; other times, it has a negative impact.

Many benign elements may bioaccumulate, meaning they do not damage or benefit organisms. While the study on these "harmless" compounds is nearly completely focused on people and lab animals, some may have a significant role in other organisms. The table below has 56 safe items. A few elements have been shown to exhibit pharmacologic action in humans. In these, a non-essential element can treat a condition (generally a micronutrient shortage). Fluorine lowers iron insufficiency.

Non-harmful radioactive elements exist. Mutations they induce affect life. This influence can be favorable or detrimental, but because mutation occurs without ionizing radiation, mutagenic compounds are not necessary for living things. All synthetic elements with atomic number 95 or higher have a limited half-life. These elements have never existed on Earth, save in tiny concentrations for brief periods. Non-biologically significant.

Aluminum is the most common metal and the third most plentiful element in Earth crust, although it is not essential to life. The eight most abundant elements in the Earth crust, which account for 90% of the crustal mass, are also essential for life.

1.2 MOLECULES OF LIFE

Biomolecules are one of the many types of compounds made by cells and other forms of life. They are also known as biological molecules and life molecules. All sorts of shapes, sizes, and functionalities may be found among biomolecules. Among biomolecules, lipids, nucleic acids, proteins, and carbohydrates are the four main types (Štefanić, 2010).

1.2.1 Carbohydrates – Sugars and Their Derivatives

The ratio of carbon (C), oxygen (O), and hydrogen (H) atoms in carbohydrates is 2:1. (As in water). Consequently, there is an empirical formula for Cm (H2O)n (where m may or may not be equal to n).

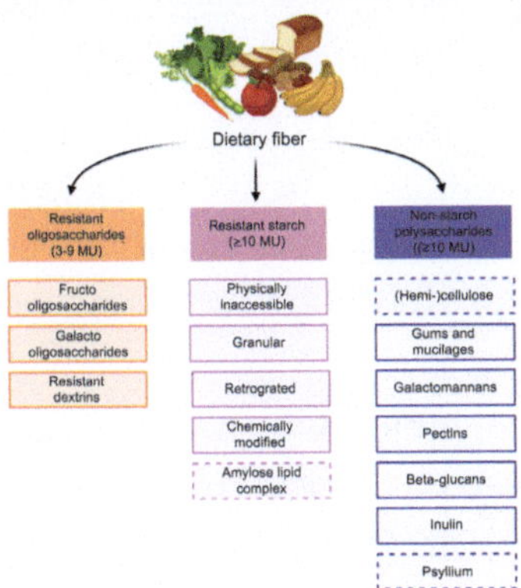

Figure 1.1: Dietary fiber food.

Source: Dietary Fibers: Effects, Underlying Mechanisms and Possible Role in Allergic Asthma Management - Scientific Figure on ResearchGate. Available from: https://www.researchgate.net/figure/Chemically-based-dietary-fiber-classification-Dietary-fibers-are-found-in-fruits_fig1_356437655 [accessed 25 Nov 2022]

In the study of biochemistry, the terms "carbohydrate" and "saccharide," which relate to sugars, starch, and cellulose, are commonly used interchangeably (Kellis, 2014).

Monosaccharides, disaccharides, oligosaccharides, and polysaccharides are the four different kinds of saccharides. The smallest (lowest molecular weight) carbohydrates are sugars, which include monosaccharides and disaccharides. In the body, carbohydrates play several important tasks. An example of a molecule with the capacity to store energy is a polysaccharide (e.g., glycogen and starch). Polysaccharides have both structural and functional purposes (e.g., chitin in arthropods and Cellulose in plants). Carbohydrates are included in many natural and manufactured foods, and they are essential to good health. Polysaccharides are what starch is categorized as. Perhaps grains could be a good source of it (wheat, maize, rice).

Carbohydrates, a kind of macromolecule, are known to the majority of individuals. "Low-carb" diets are used by some persons to lose weight. On the other side, many athletes "carb-load" in the days before a big competition to make sure they have the energy to compete at their best. Foods high in carbs, such as grains, fruits, and vegetables, are necessary for human survival. Glucose, a simple sugar, is the major source of energy from carbohydrates in the body. All living species, including people, animals, and plants, depend on carbohydrates for several additional vital functions.

A molecule with the formula (CH2O) n, where n is the number of carbon atoms in the molecule, is referred to as a carbohydrate. In other terms, the carbon to hydrogen to oxygen ratio in carbohydrate molecules is 1:2:1. The three kinds of carbohydrates are monosaccharides, disaccharides, and polysaccharides.

Glucose is the most common kind of monosaccharide (mono- = "one"; sacchar- = "sweet"). Monosaccharides are simple sugars. Monosaccharides typically have three to six carbon atoms. The prefix '-ose' is commonly used to terminate the names of monosaccharides. Trioses (three carbon atoms), Pentoses (five carbon atoms), and Hexoses (six carbon atoms) are the three categories of sugars according to the number of carbon atoms they contain (six carbon atoms). Monosaccharides can occur as a ring-shaped molecule or as a linear chain; aquatic conditions are where the ring form is most frequently seen.

The molecular formula for glucose is C6H12O6. Most living things get the majority of their energy from glucose. Glucose releases the energy needed to create adenosine triphosphate during cellular respiration (ATP). Plants produce glucose through photosynthesis using light and carbon dioxide, which is subsequently used to satisfy the demands of the plant for energy. Starch is commonly stored in place of extra glucose and is later broken down by animals that feed on plants.

Fructose and galactose are two other common monosaccharides that are both constituents of lactose or milk sugar (found in fruit). Although all three sugars share the same chemical formula (C6H12O6), their structural and chemical differences (referred to as isomers) result from differing atom locations along the carbon chain.

Disaccharides are produced when two monosaccharides (di- = "two") dehydrate (a reaction in which the removal of a water molecule occurs). When the hydroxyl group (-OH) of one monosaccharide interacts with the hydrogen atom of another monosaccharide to establish a covalent bond between the atoms of the two sugar molecules, a water molecule (H2O) is created during this process (Kellis, 2014). The disaccharides lactose, maltose, and sucrose are typical examples. Lactose is a disaccharide that is created by joining the monomers of glucose and galactose. It naturally exists in milk. The disaccharide maltose, sometimes referred to as malt sugar, is created by the transformation of two glucose molecules. The most prevalent disaccharide is sucrose, sometimes referred to as table sugar, and it is made up of the monomers glucose and fructose.

A long chain of monosaccharides joined together by covalent bonds is referred to as a polysaccharide (poly- Meaning "many"). The chain may or may not be branched and may contain different monosaccharides. Polysaccharides may comprise rather large molecules. The polysaccharides starch, glycogen, cellulose, and chitin are examples.

Sugar is stored in the plant as starch, which is made up of amylose and amylopectin (both polymers of glucose). Glucose may be produced by plants, and any extra glucose is stored as starch in several parts of the plant, including the roots and seeds. Starch is consumed by animals that then break it down into smaller molecules like glucose. The cells may then take up the glucose.

Glycogen, which is made of glucose monomers, is how humans and other creatures store glucose. The liver and muscle cells are where glycogen, the animal equivalent of starch, is normally stored. Glycogen is broken down to make glucose if blood sugar levels drop. One of the most common biopolymers to be found in nature is cellulose. Cellulose makes up the majority of the structurally supportive walls of plant cells. Cellulosic materials like wood and paper are the most common in nature. The carbon atom bonds in the glucose molecule hold the monomers that make up cellulose together.

Each additional glucose monomer in cellulose is inverted and tightly coiled into expanded, lengthy strands. Because of this, cellulose has a high tensile strength and is stiff, two qualities crucial for plant cells. A type of fiber that is digested by the body is cellulose. Although cellulose cannot be broken down by human digestive enzymes, herbivores like cows, buffaloes, and horses can digest cellulose-rich grass and use it as a food source. The rumens of these animals, which are a portion of the digestive systems of herbivores, are where the bacteria that make the cellulase enzyme live. The appendix is a crucial part of ruminant digestive tracts and also harbors bacteria that break down cellulose. The animal can utilize the glucose monomers produced by the breakdown of cellulose as a source of energy.

Carbohydrates encourage higher activity in several animals. The internal organs of arthropods, which include insects, spiders, and crabs, are shielded by their exoskeletons. The biological macromolecule chitin, a nitrogenous carbohydrate, makes up this exoskeleton. It is made up of several units of nitrogen-containing modified sugar.

The most prevalent kind of carbohydrate stored in plants is starch. Inulin is produced by several plants, including camas. Although inulin is used as a dietary fiber, some people find it difficult to digest. The flavor and texture of a raw camas bulb are unpleasant and sticky. By gently roasting camas in an underground firepit covered with certain leaves and dirt for a prolonged period, indigenous peoples make them edible and tasty. Inulin chains are transformed into ingestible mono- and disaccharides by heating. The pancreatic amylase enzyme functions similarly to this procedure (Kellis, 2014).

Camas bulbs taste similar to a cross between a baked fig and a baked pear when they are prepared properly. Despite being a food source, the blue camas should not be confused with the white death camas, which are exceedingly toxic and deadly. Although the flowers are different, the bulbs are comparable.

1.2.2 Proteins – Amino Acids

Chemical molecules known as amino acids have side chains distinct to each amino acid as well as amino and carboxylate functional groups (R group). As of 2020, more than 500 naturally occurring amino acids had been identified as monomer parts of peptides, including proteins.

The second most prevalent substance in human muscles and other tissues is protein, which is made up of amino acid residues (water being the largest). Amino acids are involved in a variety of activities, including the transport of neurotransmitters and biosynthesis, in addition to their function as protein residues. The arrangement of amino acids that make up the core structure and is the main structural component of the protein. This sequence is determined by the genetic make-up of a person. It regulates the positioning of side-chain groups along the "backbone" of a linear polypeptide (Baslé, 2010).

A protein can include up to 20 different amino acids, and the order in which they appear is very important for determining the structure and function of the protein. Proteins play a crucial role in the construction of cells. They can serve as transporters as well. The great majority of chemical processes in living things are catalyzed by enzymes and other catalysts, and nutrients and other substances are transported into and out of cells. Proteins have a role in the production of hormones and antibodies as well as the control of gene activity.

Certain amino acids, referred to as non-essential amino acids, may be produced by your body. Of the 22 amino acids, 11 are not necessary. Your body cannot manufacture any of the nine necessary amino acids. To allow your body to function properly, you must ingest enough of them. A protein is an intricate, high-molecular-weight chemical molecule comprised of peptide bonds connecting amino acids. All living cells and viruses depend on proteins for their structural and functional integrity. Enzymes or parts of enzymes are found in many proteins. Other proteins play structural or mechanical roles, such as those that build the struts and joints of the "cytoskeleton." Animals that cannot produce their energy from sunlight can still get their sustenance from proteins. The main way that proteins vary from carbohydrates is that, in addition to carbon, oxygen, and hydrogen, they also include a significant quantity of nitrogen and a very small amount of sulfur. All living things require proteins as a fundamental building block.

1.2.3 Lipids – Simple Fatty Acids

Fatty acid esters are the primary elements of biological membranes known as lipids (oleaginous). Another biological role is energy storage (e.g., triglycerides). The majority of lipids are amphiphilic because they include one to three nonpolar or hydrophobic fatty acid tails and a polar or hydrophilic head (typically glycerol). Fatty acids are unbranched chains of carbon atoms joined by single bonds (in the case of saturated fatty acids) or both single and double bonds (unsaturated fatty acids). Despite being an even number, the carbon groups in the chains frequently vary from 14 to 24.

Biological fatty acids that fall under the carboxylic acid group. At the end of a hydrocarbon chain, have one carboxyl group (COOH). Lipids are made up of a variety of distinct compounds that share a property. Lipids are hydrophobic, or "water-fearing," compounds insoluble in water because they are nonpolar molecules. This is because they are hydrocarbons that only include nonpolar carbon-carbon or carbon-hydrogen bonds. Lipids perform various functions in a cell. Cells store energy in the form of lipids known as fats for long-term use. Plants and animals are likewise insulated from their environment by lipids. They help to keep aquatic animals and birds dry because they resist water. Lipids are an important component of the plasma membrane and the building blocks of several hormones. Lipids include steroids, phospholipids, oils, and waxes.

- Saturated fatty acids: Saturated fatty acid is one kind of fatty acid (SFA). CH2 groups are connected in straight, unbranched chains by single carbon-carbon bonds. One terminal carboxylic acid group is also related to the simplest fatty acids. When a fatty acid is stated to be saturated, it indicates that every carbon atom in the chain is connected to the most hydrogen atoms. A variety of shorter-chain fatty acids have key metabolic roles. Although their chains usually include 14 to 24 carbons (Baslé, 2010).
- Unsaturated fatty acids: Unsaturated fatty acids are those that contain one or more carbon-carbon double bonds. Unsaturated molecules have fewer hydrogen atoms linked to each carbon atom than the maximum quantity. Monounsaturated compounds have one double bond, whereas polyunsaturated molecules have two or more double bonds. For example, oleic acid is a kind of monounsaturated fatty acid.
- Glycerol and cholesterol: The alcohol family includes the chemical molecule glycerol, which has a pleasant taste and is clear and colorless. Glycerides are lipids with a glycerol backbone. Glycerol is found in triglycerides, which are long-chain carboxylic acid esters of glycerol that can be derived from both plant and animal sources. In the liver and adipose tissue, glycerol serves as a precursor for the production of triacylglycerols

and phospholipids. Glycerol and fatty acids are released into circulation as the body burns stored fat for energy. Glycerol is mostly processed in the liver.

It is often utilized in FDA-approved wound and burns treatments due to its antibacterial and antiviral characteristics. The liver produces triglycerides from the building components of fatty acids and glucose. Glycerol is a glucose molecule chain. Triglycerides are formed when the chains of three fatty acids are joined together. Triglycerides are produced by both the liver and the muscles. Triglycerides are broken down to supply energy to the body when it is required. Any remaining fatty acids are carried by the blood back to the liver, where they reassociate with the glycerol chains to produce triglycerides.

Lipoproteins are two types of proteins that transport cholesterol into and out of cells. LDL, or low-density lipoprotein, is one of them. The other is HDL or high-density lipoprotein. LDL cholesterol, sometimes known as "bad" cholesterol, contributes to fatty accumulation in arteries (atherosclerosis). As a result, the arteries tighten, increasing the risk of a heart attack. A healthy amount of HDL cholesterol is regarded as "good" cholesterol because it can help avoid heart attacks and strokes.

Triglycerides are the most common kind of fat found in the body. They store whatever extra calories one ingests. High triglyceride levels have been related to fatty buildup inside the artery walls, which increases the risk of heart attack and stroke. This is especially true when paired with high LDL (bad) or low HDL (good) cholesterol levels (Kellis, 2014).

- Nucleic acids and nucleotides: Nucleic acids are found in all cells and are required for all kinds of life. Deoxyribonucleic acid (DNA) and ribonucleic acid (RNA) are the two naturally occurring forms of nucleic acids (RNA). Biopolymers are naturally occurring groupings of monomers (forming polymers) that subsequently assemble nucleotides to produce nucleic acids.

  Nucleic acids are formed when nucleotides join. These nucleotides are the building blocks of DNA. RNA and DNA are natural polymers composed of long nucleotide sequences. A nucleotide consists of a sugar molecule (ribose in RNA or deoxyribose in DNA), a phosphate group, and a nitrogen-containing base.

Adenine (A), cytosine (C), guanine (G), and thymine are the four bases utilized in DNA (T). In RNA, Uracil (U) is present in place of thymine.

Macromolecules

A macromolecule is a large molecule, such as a protein. These macromolecules are made up of thousands of atoms that are covalently bonded together. Monomers are tiny molecules that serve as the foundation for many macromolecules. A macromolecule is any exceptionally big molecule having a diameter of 100 to 10,000 angstroms (105 to 103 mm). The molecule is the smallest component of a material that has retained its qualities. A macromolecule is much bigger than a conventional molecule and has a diameter of fewer than 10 angstroms (10.06 mm) (Elias (Ed.), 2012)

Many substances, including proteins and nucleic acids, contain macromolecular components that are essential for physiology. Insulin, a protein hormone that regulates blood sugar levels, is produced by the pancreas. Its molecular building unit consists of 51 amino acids. The molecular weight of animal insulin is 5,734 g/mol.

Enzymes Act as Catalysts

Enzymes are another term for biocatalysts. They act as biological catalysts, accelerating metabolic processes in living organisms. They may be extracted from cells and utilized to catalyze a variety of processes with real-world commercial uses. The term "enzyme" was coined to describe 'the capacity of yeast to make alcohol from carbohydrates. It is derived from the Greek words en (meaning "inside") and zume (meaning "yeast").

Each enzyme contains an "active site." This place is unusual in form. A substrate is a material that an enzyme uses to perform its function. The substrate is also distinctive in form. The enzyme and the substrate must get along for the enzyme to function. Enzymes may operate as catalysts for processes without being eaten, and they only need to be present in trace amounts. The capacity of enzymes to catalyze the conversion of substrate molecules into product molecules is often expressed as follows:

Certain conditions must exist for enzymes to function properly. If the circumstances are not correct, enzymes can shift form. They do not function properly because they change form and do not fit with substrates.

Each enzyme works optimally at a certain temperature and pH. Even while proteins constitute the bulk of an enzyme, many also include a cofactor, which is a non-protein molecule. Without a cofactor, the enzyme cannot work catalytically. A cofactor can be a metal ion like iron, manganese, cobalt, copper, or zinc or an organic molecule (coenzyme).

The prosthetic group of an enzyme is a coenzyme that binds to the protein firmly and permanently. The inactive protein part of an enzyme that requires a cofactor to operate is known as an apoenzyme. This apoenzyme and a cofactor combine to form a holoenzyme (the active enzyme). Minerals and vitamins are crucial components of the human diet because they serve as cofactors and coenzymes in metabolism.

Lipids and Biomembranes

Lipids are frequently found in biological membranes, which act as barriers between cells. They divide the inside of the cell into compartments and isolate the cell from its environment. The foundation for biological membrane compartmentalization is laid by the lipid bilayer structure, which creates an impenetrable barrier for important water-soluble components in the cell. Both hydrophilic (polar) and hydrophobic (nonpolar) groups can be found in a cell molecule. As a result, the lipid constituents of the membrane are organized in a structure called a continuous bimolecular leaflet or bilayer. The nonpolar sections of the component molecules are located in the core of the bilayer, while their polar areas are located on either side of the bilayer.

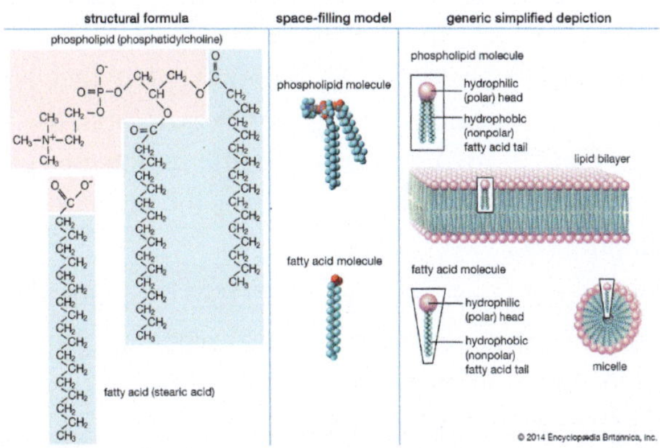

Figure 1.2: Lipids vector illustration.

Source:Thompson, 2022. Lipid. Encyclopedia Britannica. https://www.britannica.com/science/lipid

The majority of the proteins that are introduced into the bilayer create the bridge. At the point where the protein meets the nonpolar core of the lipid bilayer, membrane proteins have nonpolar side chains. Intrinsic or integral proteins are the names given to these membrane proteins. Both the polar bilayer surfaces and the intrinsic membrane proteins are related to the second group of proteins.

The containment structure of a live cell is a bilayer made of membrane lipids. Additionally, membrane lipids serve as a framework for membrane proteins. Earlier, it was believed that lipids only served a structural purpose. Lipids have several functions. They have a role in regulating cell adhesion and proliferation. They aid in the synthesis of other biomolecules. They can help enzymes become more active enzymatically.

In thylakoid membranes, monogalactosyl diglyceride, a lipid that does not form bilayers, predominates over other lipids in bulk. They develop a reverse hexagonal cylindrical phase when hydrated alone. They combine to produce lipid bilayers when combined with other lipids (Kellis, 2014).

1.3 GENES AND GENOMES

The genetic material of a cell is chemically preserved in DNA or RNA. The arrangement of the nucleotide bases in the polynucleotide chain determines the genetic instructions. A gene is a set of nucleotides that codes for a certain protein. There are hundreds of genes in the total DNA molecule of a human.

The entirety of the nuclear DNA of an organism makes up its genome. Chromosome structures are the forms in which this DNA is organized. All gene sequences are considered to be non-repetitive DNA. Numerous repeating DNA sequences make up a genome. Additionally, this repetitive DNA affects gene regulation. A gene is a specific region on a DNA molecule, but a genome is the whole nuclear DNA. This is the main difference between a gene and a genome (Hartwell, 2011).

A sequencing stretch or area on the DNA polynucleotide strand is referred to as a gene. It is regarded as the hereditary molecular unit and encodes the amino acid sequence of a particular protein. Genetic instructions are transmitted to offspring through genes.

The DNA molecule of a higher organism can have thousands of genes in it. The characters of an individual are determined by the proteins that are produced once a gene code is translated into RNA. This is the central tenet of molecular biology.

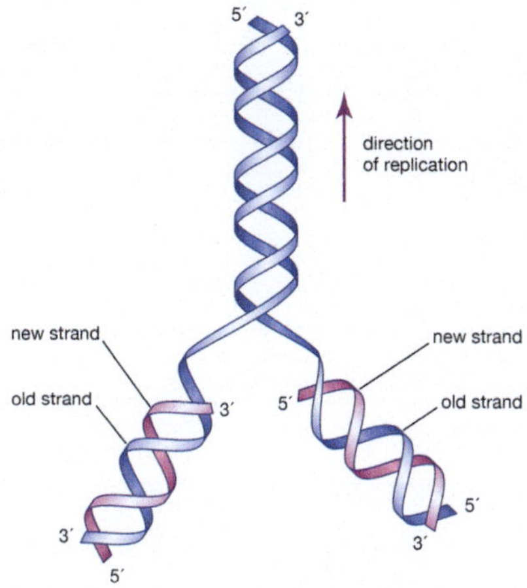

Figure 1.3: Initial proposal of DNA structure.

Source: Britannica, T. Editors of Encyclopaedia (2022, November 11). DNA. Encyclopedia Britannica. https://www.britannica.com/science/DNA

The idea of the gene and its mode of heredity was developed as a result of research in the 1860s. The study of the features of genes or gene families is known as genetics. Although a small number of genes may be constructed by RNA, DNA makes up the vast majority of genes. They are composed of RNA genes because some viruses' genetic material is RNA. In prokaryotes, clusters of genes with similar functions generate operons. Several protein-coding sequences are concurrently translated. Coding sequences and regulatory sequences make up the majority of the structure of eukaryotic genes. Introns are not present in prokaryotic genes, but exons, introns, and untranslated regions make up the coding sequence of eukaryotic genes. Gene transcription is aided by introns. They are consequently removed by exon splicing. On the other hand, alternative splicing can lead to the creation of many proteins. At both the transcriptional and translational stages, gene expression is regulated. The alternative forms of a gene are called alleles. Population phenotypic variations are caused by contrasting alleles of the same gene.

The whole nuclear DNA of an organism is referred to as its genome. Although some viruses have RNA genomes, DNA makes up the majority of viral genomes. The mitochondrial genome and chloroplast genome, respectively, are the names of respective genomes of the individual organelles. Both coding genes and non-coding junk DNA make up the genome. The complex morphology of an organism is directly correlated with its genomic size. 3.2 billion base pairs make up the human genome. Its gene count is about 25,000. Junk DNA makes up the bulk of DNA sequences in the human genome. DNA polynucleotide chains are what build each chromosome. Two sex chromosomes and 22 homologous autosome pairs make up the human genome. There are many copies of genomes of certain organisms. An organism with only one copy of its genome is said to be haploid. Multiple copies are referred to as diploid, triploid, and tetraploid. The human genome is diploid. Sexually reproducing organisms produce gametes that contain half as many chromosomes as somatic cells.

The genome of an organism is the term used to describe its genetic make-up. The whole human genome was sequenced and mapped through the Human Genome Project. Genome evolution is fueled by horizontal gene transfer and sequence duplication. Gene clusters, brief tandem repetitions, whole chromosomes, or even the whole genome can duplicate. Genomic research examines the genomes of related species (Hartwell, 2011)

1.3.1 Genes

The most basic physical and functional component of heredity is a gene. The fundamental component of genes is DNA. Some genes act as building blocks for the synthesis of proteins. However, many genes do not encode proteins. Human genes can be as little as a few hundred DNA bases or as large as 2 million bases. Humans have between 20,000 and 25,000 genes, according to the Human Genome Project, a worldwide scientific endeavor to decipher the sequence of the human genome and catalog its genes.

Every gene in a person contains two copies, one from each parent. Although a very small percentage of genes (less than 1% of the total) differ dramatically across individuals, the bulk of genes is the same in every person. Alleles are slight variations of the same gene that have different DNA base sequences. Each person has distinctive physical traits that are accentuated by these little variations.

Genes are identified by scientists by giving them distinctive names. Genes are assigned symbols, which are short string combinations of letters (and occasionally digits) that represent a condensed version of the gene name. For instance, the gene known as the cystic fibrosis transmembrane conductance regulator (CFTR) on chromosome 7 has been associated with the disease. Genes are formed of deoxyribonucleic acid (DNA), except certain viruses, which have genes made of ribonucleic acid, a molecule that is very similar to DNA (RNA). Two nucleotide strands that form a twisted ladder around one another make up a DNA molecule. The rungs of the ladder are made up of bonded pairs of nitrogenous bases, while the sides are made up of sugars and phosphates. The bases involved are adenine (A), guanine (G), cytosine (C), and thymine (T). A-T ladder rungs are created when an A on one chain connects to a T on the other; C-G ladder rungs are created when a C on one chain connects to a G on the other. The two chains unravel if the bindings of the bases are compromised, and unbound nucleotides in the cell bond to the chains' exposed bases. The free nucleotides align along each chain by the base-pairing rule; A binds to T and C binds to G. Hereditary information is passed from one cell generation to the next by this process, which splits a single original DNA molecule into two identical copies.

The arrangement of nucleotides along a strand of DNA determines the genetic code. The portion of the DNA molecule containing a particular gene divides when the product of that gene is needed. From free nucleotides in the cell, transcription creates a strand of RNA with bases matching those of the gene. Messenger RNA (mRNA), a single chain of RNA, then goes to ribosomes, organelles where translation, or protein synthesis, takes place. Transfer RNA (tRNA) lines up the nucleotides on the mRNA with specific amino acids during translation. A single amino acid is coded for by each nucleotide sequence. All proteins are made up of one or more linked polypeptide chains, which are created by a series of amino acids arranged in the sequence of nucleotides.

It has been established that not all genes produce an enzyme and that certain enzymes are made up of several small polypeptides that are produced by two or more genes. Studies have shown that many genes in animal cells are inactive for lengthy periods, if not always. So, it would seem that in both eukaryotes and prokaryotes, a gene might be switched on or off at any time. Between eukaryotes and prokaryotes, there are substantial differences in gene regulation.

It is well-accepted how genes in bacteria are activated and deactivated. The three categories of bacterial genes are the structural, operator, and regulator. The structural genes in certain polypeptides encode for their production. The DNA message of one or more structural genes is translated into mRNA by operator genes, which contain the instructions for commencing the process. As a result, structural genes and operator genes are linked together to form a functional entity called an operon. The activity of the operon is also controlled by a regulator gene that produces a small protein molecule called a repressor. The repressor binds to the operator gene and prevents it from initiating the production of the protein needed by the operon. The operon is either switched on or off depending on the presence or absence of certain repressor molecules (Hartwell, 2011).

Operon-less eukaryotic genes are independently regulated. In higher organisms, several layers of regulation are involved in the sequence of events related to gene expression, and this sequence is commonly changed by the presence or absence of molecules referred to as transcription factors. The rate of transcription is the most fundamental level of gene control, and these factors can serve as activators or enhancers. At certain periods and in particular cell types, particular transcription factors regulate the RNA that is produced from genes. The promoter, or regulatory region, found in the genes of higher organisms is commonly bound by transcription factors. Following transcription, the processes of editing and splicing remove introns (non-coding nucleotide sequences) from the primary transcript. These actions produce an active strand of mRNA. For most genes, this is a typical stage in the production of mRNA, but for certain genes, there are multiple ways to splice the original transcript, leading to diverse mRNAs, which in turn lead to different proteins. Additionally, translational and posttranscriptional regulation of certain genes exist.

A mutation happens when the number or arrangement of nucleotides in a gene is altered. Nucleotides can be added, subtracted, multiplied, shifted around, or replaced, and each modification has a distinct impact. On most creatures, a mutation has little to no impact, but when it does, the change may be harmful or even deadly. In a population, a helpful mutation will increase in frequency until it becomes the norm.

1.3.2: Genome

- Combination of recursion and mapping: The genome sequence is the whole inventory of chromosome-building nucleotides for an individual or species (A, C, G, and T for DNA genomes). Although the majority of nucleotides within a species are identical between individuals, it is important to sequence many individuals to comprehend genetic variability.

  The quantity of whole genome sequences is increasing quickly as a result of the development of new technologies that have made genome sequencing significantly less expensive and simpler. The United States National Institutes of Health manages one of the several huge genomic data databases. Rice, a mouse, *Arabidopsis thaliana*, puffer fish, and *Escherichia coli* are only a few of the thousands of organisms whose genomes have been sequenced.

In contrast to a genome sequence, which specifies the position of every DNA base in a genome, a genome map depicts landmarks. A genome map, which is less comprehensive than a genome sequence, facilitates genome-wide navigation.

- The viral genomes: The genome of a virus comprises both DNA and RNA. Genomes of RNA viruses are either single- or double-stranded and may include one or more distinct RNA molecules (segments: monopartite or multipartite genome). The majority of DNA viral genomes consist of a single, linear DNA molecule, although some are composed of circular DNA molecules.
- DNA sequences of bacterial genomes: Both prokaryotes and eukaryotes include DNA in their genomes. In contrast to archaea and the majority of bacteria, which have several linear or circular chromosomes, some bacteria carry a single circular chromosome. If DNA replication is quicker than cell division, a single bacterial cell can have many copies of a chromosome. If DNA replication is quicker than cell division, several chromosomal replications occur before cell division, allowing daughter cells to acquire both fully completed genomes and partly duplicated chromosomes. The majority of bacterial genomes include little amounts of repetitive DNA. Only around forty percent of the DNA of some symbiotic bacteria, such as *Serratia symbiotica*, which has a small genome and a high concentration of pseudogenes, encodes proteins (Hartwell, 2011).

  Some bacteria have plasmid-borne genetic material that is an integral component of their genome. Consequently, chromosomes and genomes cannot be used interchangeably.
- Eukaryotic genomes: A eukaryotic genome consists of one or more DNA chromosomes that are linear in shape. From one pair in Jack jumping ants and an asexual worm to 720 pairs in one species of fern, the number of chromosomes varies greatly. In comparison to other genomes, the amount of DNA present in eukaryotic genomes is astounding. Because the size of eukaryotic genomes may vary by up to 64,000-fold, the quantity required is substantially more than that required for DNA protein-coding and

non-coding genes. In contrast, the existence of repetitive DNA and transposable elements is what gives rise to this unique trait (TEs).

A diploid human cell has two copies of each of the 22 autosomes, one from each parent, in addition to two sex chromosomes. All gametes, including sperm, spores, and pollen, are haploid, meaning that each chromosome is present only once. DNA is also present in organelles such as chloroplasts and mitochondria, in addition to the chromosomes in the nucleus. Sometimes it is proposed that mitochondria contain their genome, known as the "mitochondrial genome." The DNA contained within chloroplasts is known as the "plastome." The circular chromosomes of mitochondria and chloroplasts are similar to those of the bacteria from whence they originated.

The exon-intron architecture of protein-coding genes is frequent in eukaryotes but rare in prokaryotes, whose genomes include variable quantities of repetitive DNA. The bulk of animal and plant genomes consist of repetitive DNA sequences. FINDER can annotate eukaryotic gene sequences.

- Coding structures: Coding sequences are DNA segments containing instructions for protein synthesis. The percentage of coding sequences inside the genome varies considerably. Larger genomes do not often include more genes, and as genome size increases in complex eukaryotes, the percentage of non-repetitive DNA decreases.

The following are some of the components that make up the human genome

- A series of introns: Introns, non-coding RNA sequences, regulatory sections, and repetitive DNA are examples of non-coding sequences. Non-coding elements constitute approximately 98% of the human genome. The genome contains two types of repetitive DNA: tandem repeats and interspersed repeats.
- Tandem repeats: Tandem repeats are short non-coding sequences that are repeated end-to-end. Minisatellites have 30 to 35 base pair repeats, while microsatellites have 2 to 5 bp repeats. Approximately 4% of the human genome and 9% of the fruit fly genome are composed of tandem repeats. The use of tandem repetitions might be advantageous. For example, mammalian

telomeres, which are essential for chromosomal end protection, consist of the tandem repeat TTAGGG.

In rare instances, an increase in tandem repetitions in exons or introns may result in illness. Typically, the human gene huntingtin (Htt) has 6-29 tandem CAG repeats (encoding a polyglutamine tract). Neurological disorder Huntington's disease is caused by an increase in the number of repetitions to greater than 36. There are twenty human disorders related to tandem repeat expansions in diverse genes. The unknown is the exact method via which proteins with enlarged polyglutamine tracts kill neurons. One idea posits that the proteins aggregate and trap essential transcription factors, impeding correct folding and influencing gene expression by preventing degradation. Replication slippage, uneven crossing-over, and gene conversion create tandem repeats.

- The capacity of components to transpose: Transposable elements (TEs) are DNA segments with a particular structure that may travel throughout the genome. There are two types of transposable elements (TEs): those that reproduce by copying and pasting, and those that may be removed from the genome and inserted elsewhere. Long interspersed nuclear elements (LINEs), interspersed nuclear elements (SINEs), and endogenous retroviruses comprise more than 45 percent of the human genome. These components can drastically affect the genetic control of an organism.

  Transport movement is an important method for genome evolution in eukaryotes since its insertion can alter gene function, homologous recombination between TEs can lead to duplications, and TE can reposition exons and regulatory sequences.

- Retrotransposons: Retrotransposons are mostly found in eukaryotes, as opposed to prokaryotes, and make up a substantial component of the genomes of many eukaryotes. A retrotransposon, a retrotransposable element, traverses an intermediary RNA molecule. Although reverse transcriptase is a specialized enzyme, retrotransposons are composed of DNA but are first transcribed into RNA before being replicated back into DNA. Retrotransposons with reverse transcriptase can initiate their transposition, but those without the enzyme must rely on reverse transcriptase produced by another retrotransposon.

Retrotransposons are capable of being translated into RNA and then copied to a new location on the genome. Long terminal repeats (LTRs), and non-long terminal repeats (NLTRs) are the two forms of retrotransposons (non-LTRs).

Non-long terminal repeats (non-LTRs) are divided into three distinct categories: long interspersed nuclear elements (LINEs), short interspersed nuclear elements (SINEs), and Penelope-like elements (PLEs). There are a greater number of DIRS-like Non-LTR components in the bacterium *Dictyostelium discoideum*. Non-LTRs are prevalent in the genomes of eukaryotes (Hartwell, 2011).

Long interspersed elements (LINEs) are autonomous transposable elements because they contain genes for reverse transcriptase and endonuclease. Approximately 500,000 LINEs make up 17% of the human genome. Short interspersed elements (SINEs) rely on the proteins encoded by LINEs for transposition since they are non-autonomous and have less than 500 base pairs on average

- DNA transposons: Between inverted terminal repeats, DNA transposons include an enzyme called transposase. When the transposase is produced, it identifies the terminal inverted repeats of the transposon and initiates the excision and reinsertion at a new location. This strategy usually introduces transposons close to their point of origin (within 100 kb). DNA transposons, which are also present in bacteria, constitute 3% of the human genome and 11% of the genome of *Caenorhabditis elegans*.

Dimensions of the Genome

The number of identified proteins in genomes submitted to GenBank is depicted on a log-log plot based on genome size. The total amount of DNA base pairs in a single copy of a haploid genome. The size of the genome of each species varies considerably. Small-genome invertebrates contain fewer transposable elements. Compared to fish and amphibians, birds have relatively tiny genomes; nonetheless, it is believed that birds lost a significant amount of their genomes when they developed to fly. Before this loss, DNA methylation permits proper genome development.

The human nuclear genome consists of 24 linear molecules totaling 3.1 billion nucleotides, with the shortest chromosome containing 45 million nucleotides and the longest chromosome including 248 million nucleotides.

In neither prokaryotes nor lower eukaryotes is there a clear and consistent relationship between morphological complexity and genome size. The growth and contraction of repetitive DNA components have a significant effect on the size of the genome.

Genome Evolution

Genomes have features that may be analyzed and investigated independently of the specifics of any given gene and its effects; they are more than just the genetic content of an organism. Researchers evaluate characteristics such as karyotype (chromosome number), genome size, gene order, codon usage bias, and GC content to establish the mechanisms that may have contributed to the formation of the wide array of genomes that exist today. Duplications serve a crucial part in the formation of the genome.

There are several kinds of duplication, ranging from the expansion of small tandem repeats to the duplication of a group of genes to the duplication of entire chromosomes and even complete genomes. It is considered that these duplications are crucial to the evolution of genetic innovation.

Horizontal gene transfer is the cause of the remarkable similarity between small portions of the genomes of two species that are otherwise distantly related. It indicates that horizontal gene transfer is prevalent among microorganisms. In addition, it appears that mitochondrial and chloroplast genomes were transferred to nuclear chromosomes in eukaryotic cells.

CHAPTER 2

HISTORY OF BIOINFORMATICS

CONTENTS

2.1: INTRODUCTION

Students and researchers nowadays typically assume that recent advances in bioinformatics have facilitated the processing of next-generation sequencing data. Bioinformatics began more than 60 years ago when desktop computers were there but the DNA sequencing technology was not yet available. The use of computer technologies for protein sequence analysis in the early 1960s created the groundwork for bioinformatics. Later advances in computer science and molecular biology made it easier to alter and sequence DNA, paving the way for DNA analysis. From the 1990s to the 2000s, a massive rise in sequencing technology and declining costs led to an exponential explosion of data. The introduction of "Big Data" has necessitated the incorporation of additional computer scientists due to the emergence of new issues in data mining and administration. Biological Big Data has (and continues to have) considerable implications on the predictive power and repeatability of bioinformatics results when combined with a growing collection of bioinformatics tools. To address this issue, institutions are now completely integrating this subject into their biology curriculum. Synthetic biology, systems biology, and whole-cell modeling are recent sub-disciplines of biology that have emerged as a result of the increased interaction between computer science and biology (Gauthier, 2019).

Biologists' arsenals now include computers and sophisticated software. Computers are used in virtually all current biology research initiatives, whether for ordinary DNA or protein sequence analysis or for analyzing significant information in gigabyte-sized biological data sets. This is especially true now that next-generation sequencing (NGS) has substantially altered a vast array of scientific domains, including population genetics, quantitative genetics, molecular systematics, microbial ecology, and many more.

In this setting, it is easy for students and researchers to assume that current bioinformatics is a recent innovation that has facilitated the interpretation of NGS data. Bioinformatics began more than 50 years ago when desktop computers were, but a concept and DNA sequencing was not yet available. We give a complete chronology of important breakthroughs in bioinformatics and related topics during the past fifty years, in addition to some background on contemporaneous improvements in molecular biology and computer science and some projections for the future of the subject. This overview should help the reader understand why bioinformatics has assumed such an important role in biology. Since the identification of 579 human genes in 1981, *in situ* hybridization mapping has been more popular. The automated DNA sequencing method developed by Marvin Carruthers and

Leroy Hood is a significant achievement in bioinformatics. Human Genome Organization (HUGO) was created in 1988. This international association comprises Human Genome Project scientists. The first exhaustive genetic map of the *Haemophilus influenza* bacterium was published in 1989. The Human Genome Project began the next year. In 1991, a total of 1879 human genes were identified. In 1993, the French Center for Research on the Human Genome, Genethon, developed a physical map of the human genome. Genethon released the final version of 'The Human Genetic Map' three years later. At this moment, the first phase of the 'Human Genome Project' concluded. GenBank, EMBL, and the Japanese DNA Database were created to preserve and compare DNA sequence data generated by the human genome and other genome sequencing efforts. Bioinformatics is gradually incorporating protein structure analysis, gene and protein functional data, patient data, pre-clinical and clinical investigations, and metabolic pathways from other species (Gauthier, 2019).

2.2 1950–1970: THE ORIGINS

At the beginning of the 1950s, little was known about deoxyribonucleic acid (DNA). At the time, its role as a molecule that transfers genetic information was still up for question. Avery, MacLeod, and McCarty (1944) proved that taking pure DNA from a virulent bacterial strain may transfer virulence to a nonvirulent strain; however, their findings were not immediately accepted by the scientific community. Many folks believed that proteins carried genetic information. In 1952, Hershey and Chase demonstrated beyond a reasonable doubt that bacterial cells infected with a bacteriophage took up and transferred DNA rather than protein, establishing the significance of DNA as a molecule containing genetic information.

Despite its critical function, the structure of the DNA molecule was little understood. It was only known that its monomers (i.e., nucleotides) were present in equal amounts. The amounts of adenosine, thymidine, guanidine, and cytidine are equal. In 1953, Watson, Crick, and Franklin successfully determined the DNA double-helix structure. Despite this discovery, it would need a further 13 years to understand the genetic code and 25 years to develop the first DNA sequencing technique. As a result, bioinformatics applications for DNA analysis trailed behind those for proteins by around 20 years, as the chemical composition of proteins was previously more thoroughly understood than that of DNA (Gauthier, 2019).

Protein Analysis Was the Starting Point

The first insulin amino acid sequence or arrangement was published in the late 1950s, coinciding with significant advances in the capacity of crystallography to detect protein structures. Because of this crucial finding, the problem of protein polypeptide chain production was ultimately solved. It also aided in the development of more effective methods for collecting protein sequences. The Edman degradation was developed as a simple technique for sequencing proteins, starting at the N-terminus and working up to the C-terminus. Over the next ten years, automated sequencing was used to sequence over 15 distinct protein families.

Obtaining long protein sequences was a significant difficulty for Edman sequencing. Edman sequencing cleaves N-terminal amino acid residues one at a time using phenylisothiocyanate. However, this reaction never yields a finished product. As a result, the only way to create a sequence of 50 to 60 amino acids is by an Edman reaction. Smaller pieces of bigger proteins must first be isolated before sequencing.

It was more difficult to reassemble the whole protein sequence from millions of tiny Edman peptide sequences than it was to sequence a protein. It takes some time to obtain the whole sequence of big proteins having hundreds of thousands of amino acids. To address this issue, one of the earliest known bioinformatics software systems was created in the early 1960s.

Dayhoff: The First Bioinformaticians

Margaret Dayhoff (1925–1983) was a pioneer in the use of computational approaches to biochemistry. Former National Center for Biotechnology Information director David J. Lipman has referred to the contributions of Dayhoff to this discipline as "the mother and father of bioinformatics" (NCBI).

'The Ph.D. thesis of Dayhoff in electrochemistry made extensive use of computational approaches, and she saw the promise of computers in biology and medicine. In 1960, she was appointed associate director of the National Biomedical Resource Foundation. Robert S. Ledley, a physicist who shared her interest in using computer technology for medical problems, became her employer. Between 1958 and 1962, they collaborated to develop COMPROTEIN, a "full computer software for the IBM 7090" that predicted the primary structure of proteins using Edman peptide sequencing data. This software is the earliest example of what we now call a de novo sequence assembler, and it was created entirely in FORTRAN using punch cards. Input and output amino acid sequences of the COMPROTEIN software were identified by three-letter acronyms (e.g., Lys for lysine, Ser for serine). To improve the storing of protein sequence data, Dayhoff later created the one-letter amino acid code, which is still in use today. The first biological sequence database ever developed, Dayhoff and Eck's Atlas of Protein Sequence and Structure, was published in 1965 with this one-letter identifier. The original edition of the Atlas had 65 protein sequences, the majority of which were interspecific variations of a few proteins. Since it is believed that protein sequences preserve the evolutionary history of species, the first Atlas provided the ideal data set for two scientists to verify their hypothesis (Gauthier, 2019).

The Computer-Assisted Genealogy of Life

Before the 1960s, the majority of biochemistry research focused on enzyme mechanistic modeling. Emile Zuckerkandl and Linus Pauling, on the other hand, deviated from this paradigm by seeing biomolecular sequences as "information carriers." The organization of amino acids of a protein into a "word" determines its molecular function (i.e., meaning), similar to how words are created from sequences of letters whose order provides meaning. Protein sequences, like words and languages, can develop through the delayed inheritance of minute changes. Could we utilize these genetic differences to retrace the evolution of these proteins and their "ancestor" sequence? Paleogenetics was coined by Zuckerkandl and Pauling in 1963 to describe a young discipline of evolutionary biology.

Both investigations discovered that the degree of similarity between orthologous proteins from vertebrate species, including hemoglobin, was far too high to be the result of chance or convergent evolution through time (Ibid). Walter M. Fitch founded orthology in 1970 to detect homology stemming from a speciation event. Furthermore, it was shown that the degree of variation between orthologs from various species is connected to evolutionary divergence. Human hemoglobin, for example, resembled chimp hemoglobin (Pan Troglodytes) more than mouse (*Mus musculus*) hemoglobin. This gradient in sequence identity was compatible with fossil-based divergence estimates.

Based on these facts, Zuckerkandl and Pauling proposed that orthologous proteins evolved from a common ancestor. By analyzing hemoglobin sequences in extant species, it was possible to determine the "ancestral sequences" of hemoglobin and, as a result, its evolutionary history up to its current forms.

Nonetheless, there were several conceptual and computational challenges to solve, the most notable of which was assessing the "evolutionary value" of protein sequence changes. A second issue was the lack of effective methods for aligning protein sequences. An early sequence-based phylogenetic investigation of proteins led to the discovery of homologs from different mammalian species that were so similar that a visual comparison of only a few sites was enough to infer similarity. For proteins with a more distant origin or with varying sequence lengths, this procedure may be difficult or lead to incorrect findings (Gauthier, 2019)

Needleman and Wunsch devised the first dynamic programming approach for pairwise protein sequence alignments in 1970, which helped greatly to the solution of this challenge. Despite this considerable breakthrough, the first multiple sequence alignment (MSA) approach did not appear until the early 1980s. The original MSA approach, a Needleman-Wunsch variant, used a scoring matrix with the same number of dimensions as the number of sequences. The computational complexity of this MSA approach is O (LN), where L is the length of the sequence, and N is the number of sequences. To accurately align 10 sequences of 100 residues each, 1018 operations are required or the sequence length multiplied by the number of sequences. Using this method would make aligning hundreds of proteins of varying lengths challenging.

Da-Fei Feng and Russell F. Doolitle identified the first fully viable treatment for MSA in 1987. Needleman-Wunsch alignments are performed on each pair of sequences, pairwise similarity scores are acquired, a guide tree is created using the scores, and the two most similar sequences are aligned first, followed by the next most similar sequences, and so on. CLUSTAL, a popular MSA program developed in 1988 to simplify the Feng-Doolittle approach, is still in use today (Gauthier, 2019).

A Mathematical Framework for Amino Acid Substitutions

Dayhoff, Schwartz, and Orcutt created the first probabilistic model of amino acid substitutions in 1978, contributing to another bioinformatics milestone. The discovery of 1572 point accepted mutations (PAMs) in the evolutionary trees of 71 protein families with greater than 85 percent similarity served as the basis for this model, which was finished eight years after it was initiated. The result was a 20-20 asymmetric substitution matrix with probability values based on observed amino acid changes (i.e., the probability that each amino acid will change in a given small evolutionary interval). Previously, in phylogenetic reconstructions, the idea (i.e., minimum number of changes) was employed to quantify evolutionary distance; however, the PAM matrix includes the notion of substitutions as a measure of evolutionary change.

Significant advancements in molecular biology, meantime, have transformed DNA into the principal reservoir of biological information. Following the discovery of the chemical composition of the DNA and its role as a gene carrier, it became evident that DNA would hold an astounding amount of biological information.

Deciphering the DNA Language: The Genetic Code

The DNA molecule encodes the properties of every living entity through its unique nucleotide sequences (more precisely, its "proteins"). This viewpoint was formalized by the sequence hypothesis of Francis Crick (now known as the "Central Dogma"), which proposed that RNA sequences translated from DNA determine the amino acid sequence of the proteins they produce. The three-dimensional structure of a protein is dictated by the amino acid sequence.

By determining how the cell turns the "DNA language" into polypeptide sequences, one can "read" the DNA of an organism and anticipate the fundamental structure of every protein it creates. By 1968, all 64 codons of the genetic code had been decoded, becoming DNA "readable." This astounding discovery demanded the development of rapid, low-cost technology for gathering DNA sequences (Huang, J. 2022).

Cost-efficient Reading of DNA

In 1976, the Maxam-Gilbert sequencing method was the first to acquire general recognition. The laboratory approach of Frederick Sanger practically precludes its use due to the intensive use of radiation and poisonous chemicals, as well as its inherent complexity. In 1977, 25 years after discovering the first protein sequence, Sanger's team developed the "plus and minus" DNA sequencing method, which was the first to use primed synthesis using DNA polymerase. This method was used to sequence the genome of the bacteriophage X174 (5,386 base pairs), the first DNA genome ever discovered. The popular Sanger chain termination method, which is still in use forty years later, was established as a result of technological breakthroughs in "plus and minus" DNA sequencing.

Collecting DNA sequences from a single organism leads to several information throughput gains. In contrast to proteins, which must be purified individually before sequencing, it is feasible to get the whole genome of an organism from a single genomic DNA extract. This DNA sequence of the whole genome may be used to predict the primary structure of all proteins made by an organism via gene translation. Despite its apparent simplicity, manual extraction of information from DNA sequences entails the following steps:

1. Comparisons (for example, determining homology across sequences from different species);
2. Calculations (for example, using the PAM1 matrix to generate a phylogenetic tree with numerous protein orthologs)

In some tasks, computers are significantly more efficient and productive than people. Dayhoff and Eck proved that computer-assisted protein sequence analysis gave more information than mechanistic modeling alone; similarly, the extraordinary readability of the DNA sequence needed a comparable study technique.

In 1979, Roger Staden created the first tool to analyze the findings of Sanger sequencing. (I) look for overlaps in Sanger gel readings. The Staden Package was one of the first sequence analysis tools that employs additional characters to indicate base calling errors in a sequence read. The current International Union of Biochemistry and Molecular Biology (IUBMB) nomenclature for nucleic acid sequences with poorly defined bases was inspired by this enlarged DNA alphabet. The Staden Package is still under construction (Huang, J. 2022)

Using DNA Sequences in Phylogenetic Inference

Ernst Haeckel proposed certain notions linked to phylogeny in 1866, but the earliest molecular phylogenetic trees were constructed from protein sequences and assumed maximum parsimony (i.e., the fewest number of changes) to be the primary mechanism driving evolutionary change. According to the 1981 remark of Joseph Felsenstein on parsimony-based techniques, they initially assume that change is unlikely (Felsenstein 1973, 1979). If there are little differences between the examined phases of evolution, parsimony approaches will be useful statistical tools. When the bulk of data demonstrates moderate to considerable quantities of change, parsimony strategies may fail.In addition, selection, mutation, and random mutation all influence the evolution of the genes that encode proteins. Nucleic acid sequencing supplied phylogenetics with the knowledge that amino acid sequencing did not. Due to the degeneracy of the genetic code, synonymous mutations (a nucleotide substitution that does not alter the amino acids) may only be discovered using nucleotide sequences as input. Felsenstein devised the maximum likelihood (ML) technique for reconstructing phylogenetic trees from DNA sequences. In contrast to parsimony approaches, which utilize the fewest number of alterations to reconstruct an evolutionary tree, ML estimation "involves identifying the evolutionary tree that provides the best probability of evolving the provided data."

As a result of the research by Felsenstein on molecular phylogeny, several ML-based bioinformatics tools have been developed and are continually being enhanced. Additionally, new statistical methods for evaluating the resilience of nodes have been created. This led to the widespread use of Bayesian statistics in molecular phylogeny in the 1990s, which are still widely employed in modern biology.

Late in the 1970s, significant technological obstacles had to be surmounted to expand the use of computers in DNA analysis (not to mention DNA analysis itself). The subsequent decade was crucial for overcoming these obstacles (Gauthier, 2019).

2.3 1980–1990: PARALLEL ADVANCES IN BIOLOGY AND COMPUTER SCIENCE

Molecular Methods to Target and Amplify Specific Genes

Genes cannot be biochemically isolated from proteins and RNAs before being individually sequenced since they are all located on a tiny number of DNA molecules per cell. Moreover, each cell normally has one too many copies of a gene. Thus, genes are orders of magnitude rarer than the proteins they encode.

In the approach followed by Jackson, Symons, and Berg (1972) approach, circular SV40 viral DNA was cut and introduced into lambda DNA using restriction endonucleases and DNA ligase before being utilized to convert *Escherichia coli* cells. As the inserted DNA molecule replicates in the host organism and is amplified in *E. coli* cells, millions of copies of a single DNA insert are created. This study was a pioneer in gene isolation and amplification independent of the original organism (for instance, SV40 is a virus that infects primates). Berg called for a prohibition on the use of recombinant DNA because he was concerned about the possible ethical difficulties (eugenics, warfare, and unforeseen biological dangers). Berg presided over the 1975 Asilomar summit when a set of genetic standards that are still in use today were defined.

The second significant breakthrough in DNA manipulation was the polymerase chain reaction (PCR), which allows DNA amplification without the requirement for cloning techniques. Kjell Kleppe et al. published the first "repair synthesis" using DNA polymerase in 1971; nonetheless, Kary Mullis is credited with developing PCR due to his significant improvements to this technique (notably the use of the thermostable Taq polymerase and development of the thermal cycler). Mullis gained the greatest credit for developing PCR because, unlike Kleppe and others, he patented his invention.

Increasingly, gene cloning and PCR are utilized to generate DNA libraries, which are required to collect sequence information. Due to the discovery of DNA sequencing in the late 1970s and improved DNA manipulation, a rising quantity of sequence data is currently accessible. In the 1980s, the availability of computers and bioinformatics software increased.

Access to Computers and Specialized Software

Before the 1970s, a "minicomputer" was equivalent in size and weight to a small domestic refrigerator, omitting the terminal and storage units. Due to the size restriction, it was difficult for individuals or small organizations to purchase computers. Even after the introduction of the 8080 microprocessor of Intel in 1974, early desktop computers lacked user-friendliness, with many systems (such as the Altair 8800) requiring the operating system to be loaded manually through binary switches upon startup (Huang, J. 2022)

The year 1977 marked the introduction of the first fully working microcomputers to the consumer market. The Commodore PET, Apple II, and Tandy TRS-80, the first three computers in this wave, were compact, affordable, and user-friendly at the time. Each of the three contained a BASIC interpreter, a user-friendly language for non-programmers.

Rapidly, biology-related software was developed. The year 1984 saw the publication of the "GCG" software package by the University of Wisconsin Genetics Computer Group. The GCG package contains 33 command-line utilities for altering DNA, RNA, and protein sequences. The GCG package was created to operate on a fundamental mainframe system. This was the first software program created for sequence analysis.

In the same year as GCG, another sequence manipulation suite was developed. In the 1980s and 1990s, DNASTAR, a software package that ran on CP/M personal computers and could compile and analyze Sanger sequencing data, gained popularity. More sequence manipulation applications for CP/M, Apple II, and Macintosh computers were created in 1984 and 1985. Some of the software developers provided free copies of the source code upon request, foreshadowing an upcoming trend in the programming world of software sharing (Gauthier, 2019).

Bioinformatics and the Free Software Movement

Richard Stallman wrote the GNU Manifesto in 1985, in which he stated his rationale for developing the free operating system GNU (Not Unix of GNU). This movement eventually gave rise to the Free Software Foundation, which advocates the notion that "users have the right to run, copy, distribute, study, alter, and improve the software." Other bioinformatics projects, such as the European Molecular Biology Open Software Suite, which began development as a free and open-source alternative to GCG later in 1996, were based on 'the free software concept of Stallman. Before the GNU project, other initiatives displayed this line of thinking. The macromolecular X-ray crystallography Collaborative Computational Project Number 4 (CCP4), which began in 1979 and is still widely utilized, is one such example.

The European Molecular Biology Laboratory (EMBL), GenBank, and DNA Data Bank of Japan (DDBJ) sequence databases converged at this time to standardize data formatting, determine the minimal information for reporting nucleotide sequences, and permit data interchange across those databases. This is of considerable importance. The year 1986 saw the merger of EMBL and GenBank, followed by DDBJ in 1987. Currently, the International Nucleotide Sequence Database Collaboration represents this union, which is still in existence.

Throughout the 1980s, bioinformatics developed sufficient popularity in modern study to merit its publication. The bioinformatics magazine Computer Applications in the Biosciences (CABIOS) was founded in 1985 in response to the growing availability of computers and the vast potential for computer-assisted analysis in biological fields. This publication, now known as Bioinformatics, was tasked with democratizing bioinformatics among scientists.

CABIOS is a publication for life scientists interested in learning how computers might improve their jobs. Emphasis is placed on application and its solid scientific foundation. Undoubtedly, there is a need for a publication that provides in-depth evaluations and research that give the terminology, terms of reference, and conceptual framework for all elements of biological computing. Computing should not be more mysterious than any other scientific method.

The emergence of specialized scientific publications and the rise of the free software movement contributed to a growth in the use of computers in biology. For enormous data collections, such as whole genomes and gene catalogs, however, small-scale mainframe computers were utilized rather than microcomputers. These systems usually made use of Unix-like operating systems and languages different than those used on microcomputers, such as FORTRAN and C. (such as BASIC and Pascal). Popular sequence analysis software designed for microcomputers was not necessarily compatible with mainframe systems, and *vice versa* (Huang, J. 2022)

Desktop Computers and New Programming Languages

With the emergence of x86 and RISC microprocessors in the early 1980s, a new type of personal computer arose. Desktop workstations have proportions comparable to those of microcomputers but much superior hardware performance and software architecture like that of mainframe computers. They were created for scientific and technological uses. Indeed, desktop workstations were typically powered by Unix-based operating systems and their variants, such as HP-UX and BSD.

Several scripting languages that are still frequently used by bioinformaticists today emerged in the mid-1980s. These programming languages use natural language qualities to facilitate the writing of programs while abstracting essential components of computer systems. Scripted applications typically do not need to be compiled because they are interpreted as soon as they are launched, albeit running more slowly than identical C or Fortran programs.

Perl (Practical Extraction and Reporting Language) was developed by Larry Wall in 1987 as a GNU operating system extension to ease text data processing and reporting. Perl is a multiparadigm, high-level, interpreted programming language. Because biological sequence data can be easily saved in text format, it is the appropriate language for manipulating this sort of data. The first Perl-based bioinformatics software was created in 1994. Because of its versatility, Perl was the industry standard for bioinformatics until the late 2000s. According to Larry Wall, there are various ways to accomplish it. The 1996 introduction of BioPerl elevated the status of Perl in the field of bioinformatics (and its initial release in 2002). The modules in this Perl programming interface aid with routine yet difficult operations, such as obtaining sequence data from nearby and distant databases, II switching between file formats, III doing similarity searches, and IV annotating sequence data.

However, the flexibility of Perl and often punctuated syntax can rapidly result in illegible code. Because of this, it may be difficult to maintain Perl code, particularly when updating software that has been in use for some time. At the same time, another high-level programming language was poised to play a key role in the bioinformatics business.

In 1989, Guido van Rossum developed Python, an additional multiparadigm, high-level programming language. Python was designed to have a simpler vocabulary and grammar to improve code readability and maintenance, notwithstanding the potential of equivalent applications for both languages (at the sacrifice of versatility). However, it was not until the year 2000 that dedicated Python bioinformatics libraries were developed, and it was not until the late 2000s that Python became a prominent programming language in the discipline. In the early 1990s, other non-scripting programming languages, such as Perl and Python, emerged and eventually made their way into the bioinformatics field.

Since the early 1990s, increasingly complicated operations, such as the study of whole genomes from prokaryotic and eukaryotic species, have been made feasible by the advent of *in vitro* or *in silico* tools for DNA analysis (Gauthier, 2019).

2.4 1990–2000: GENOMICS, STRUCTURAL BIOINFORMATICS, AND THE INFORMATION SUPERHIGHWAY

Dawn of the Genomics Era

In 1995, the researcher J. The Institute for Genomic Research (TIGR), directed by Craig Venter, sequenced the first complete genome of a free-living organism (*Haemophilus influenzae*). However, the age of genomics as we know it now started with the publishing of the human genome at the turn of the twenty-first century. The Human Genome Project was begun by the National Institutes of Health in 1991, and its 13-year lifespan cost taxpayers $2.7 billion (in 1991 money). In 1998, Venter's biotechnology business, Celera Genomics, initiated a private, competitive attempt to read and assemble the human genome. The Celera-funded initiative successfully sequenced and assembled the human genome at a quarter of the cost of the NIH-funded research. The utilization of NIH data by Celera-led research and the employment of distinct experimental methods resulted in a tenfold disparity between public and private effort costs.

Despite scientific optimism, whole-genome sequencing takes millions of dollars and years to complete, even for a bacterial genome. Currently, sequencing the human genome would cost $1,000 and require less than a week. Even though numerous library preparation methods were available at the time, Sanger capillary sequencers were employed to collect sequencing reads, which explains the substantial cost difference. With a maximum throughput of just 96 reads of 800 bp per run, they were orders of magnitude slower than second-generation sequencers from the late 2000s. To get one-fold coverage, it is necessary to sequence the human genome (3.0 Gbp) at least 40,000 times.

In addition to the tedious laboratory methods, specialized software must be developed to manage this enormous amount of data. In the middle to late 1990s, PHRAP, Celera Assembler, TIGR Assembler, MIRA, EULER, and others were designed to assemble whole-genome sequencing reads using Perl.

In the early years of genomics, the global information network, which emerged in the early 1990s, had a crucial role. The NIH-funded human genome sequencing project makes its data publicly accessible via this network of networks. This network would rapidly grow throughout the scientific community, notably for data and software exchange.

Bioinformatics Online

The contributions of Tim Berners During his time as a researcher at the Conseil Européen de Recherche Nucléaire (CERN) in the early 1990s, Lee developed the World Wide Web, a worldwide information system comprised of linked sites. Since the mid-1990s, the Internet has altered culture, business, and technology, allowing humans to interact practically immediately for the first time in history. (Wishart, D. S. (Eds.). 2020). This technique resulted in the development of internationally accessible bioinformatics resources. In 1993, the EMBL Nucleotide Sequence Data Library was the first nucleotide sequence database to be made available over the World

Wide Web. It includes several other databases, such as SWISS-PROT and REBASE. In 1992, nearly simultaneously, the NCBI gained management of the GenBank database (before it was under contract with Los Alamos National Laboratory). However, GenBank was not always accessible online; it was initially released on CD-ROM and in print.

In 1994, the well-known NCBI website was also made available online. (Includes the Basic Local Alignment Search Tool, or BLAST tool, which enables rapid completion of pairwise alignments). Several major databases that are still in use today, including Genomes, PubMed, and Human Genome, were subsequently built (Wishart, D. S. (Eds.). 2020).

Access to bioinformatics tools has been widened and simplified by the proliferation of Web resources, particularly via the use of Web servers with intuitive graphical user interfaces. Even for experienced bioinformaticians, (i) bioinformatics software frequently requires prior knowledge of UNIX-like operating systems, (ii) requires the use of command lines (for both installation and usage), and (iii) requires the installation of multiple software libraries (dependencies) before use.

Thankfully, more developers are striving to make their products accessible to the scientific community via simple graphical Web servers, allowing data analysis without the need for time-consuming installation processes. These days, web servers are utilized so often in research that an annual special issue of the journal Nucleic Acids Research is devoted to them.

In addition to data analysis, the Internet also served as a platform for the dissemination of scientific works through publication. Since The Philosophical Transactions of the Royal Society, the earliest scientific journal, was created in 1665, scientists have disseminated their findings through written and spoken channels.

In the early 1980s, many examinations into the practicality, benefits, and drawbacks of utilizing the Internet for scientific publication commenced (including submission, revision, and reading of articles). BLEND, a three-year research project involving over fifty scientists, was one of the early efforts to shed light on the possibilities and difficulties of such systems. These were the first research to post and archive data online. This se is evidenced by the installation of multitasking preprint servers such as arXiv from Cornell University and bioRxiv of Cold Spring Harbor (2013).

Beyond Sequence Analysis: Structural Bioinformatics

The three-dimensional structure of myoglobin was established by X-ray diffraction in 1958. In 1951, Pauling and Corey published two studies predicting -helices and -sheets, laying the groundwork for protein structure prediction. Because of fold recognition algorithms, also known as treading, it is now possible to determine the secondary and tertiary structure of proteins with varying degrees of precision using computers.

Although advances in 3D structure prediction are critical, it is important to remember that proteins are dynamic networks of atoms rather than static structures. Force fields that characterize the interactions between atoms made it feasible to mimic the molecular dynamics of proteins as a result of biophysical advancements in the 1990s. Despite the development of tools and theoretical techniques, molecular dynamics simulations are difficult to accomplish in practice due to the high computer resource needs. Even with supercomputers with 256 central processing units, it took months in 1998 to model a 36-amino acid peptide (villin headpiece subdomain) in a microsecond.

Despite the constant development in computer processing power, many biomolecules are still unable to run molecular dynamics simulations on a realistic time scale due to a lack of computing resources. However, several developments have occurred and continue to occur that make molecular dynamics more accessible, such as the use of graphics processing units (GPUs) via high-performance graphics cards, which are commonly used for graphics or video games. Furthermore, the use of GPUs expanded to other areas of bioinformatics that needed significant processing capability, such as the development of molecular phylogenies.

However, the ease with which data can be released over the Internet, along with the increase in computing power, has resulted in the fast proliferation of information known as "Big Data" (Gauthier, 2019).

2.5 2000–2010: HIGH-THROUGHPUT BIOINFORMATICS

Second-Generation Sequencing

With the advent of second-generation sequencing, also known as next-generation sequencing or NGS, which began with the '454' pyrosequencing process, DNA sequencing became more affordable. This method restored the former computational constraint by enabling the sequencing of hundreds of thousands to millions of DNA molecules in a single machine cycle. The proprietary tool Newbler, which Roche maintained until the 454 was discontinued in 2016, remains the gold standard for handling 454 readings (high-throughput sequencer). There are presently a great deal more firms, technologies, and methods available to manage sequences.

Currently, there are so many tools available that it is impossible to choose just one. If this trend continues, it may become increasingly difficult for various study teams to compare and reproduce the findings of one another. Since transferring to newer and/or alternative bioinformatics tools requires more training and testing, researchers are hesitant to abandon the software they are accustomed to. Therefore, the justification for acquiring new abilities must be an improvement in computation time or notably superior results. Consequently, contests, such as the well-known Assemblathon, which assesses de novo assemblers based on performance measures, have evolved. However, the rise of accessible technology is dwarfed by the exponential growth of biological data stored in open databases.

Biological Big Data

Moore's Law was no longer an accurate predictor of future costs after the 2008 introduction of massively parallel sequencing technology when the cost of DNA sequencing plummeted by many orders of magnitude. As a result, the number of sequences in public databases like GenBank and WGS increased enormously, as did interest in big data concerns. In reality, the scientific community has already created data that exceeds the Exabyte (1018) threshold. It takes a lot of computing power to manage all this data, not only to store it but also to arrange it for easy access and usage. (Wishart, D. S. (Eds.). 2020). New repository infrastructure has emerged for model species, such as Drosophila, Saccharomyces, and humans. In addition to genomic sequences with annotations (often curated) and metadata, a significant number of these specialist databases also include tools for researchers investigating these organisms. Dicty Stock Center, a directory of strains and plasmids, is a handy supplement to dictyBase, a database of the model organism *Dictyostelium discoideum*. The Sequence Read Archive and the European Nucleotide Archive, which were created to archive raw sequencing data for enhanced research repeatability, have also gained in popularity.Given the growing number of genetic sequences and databases, it is vital to establish criteria for organizing these new resources, ensuring their long-term survival, and allowing their usage. The Genomic Standards

Consortium was founded in 2005 to determine the absolute minimum of data required for a genomic sequence (Gauthier, 2019).

High-Performance Bioinformatics and Collaborative Computing

The increase in bioinformatics initiatives and the escalating volume of data have compelled financial authorities to take action. Similar to the vast majority of scientific investigations, bioinformatics projects require financing.

The computer is the most prevalent instrument utilized in bioinformatics research. Even though a simple desktop computer may be utilized in some instances and for some computations, many bioinformatics projects may require infrastructures that are far more complex, costly, and require specialist knowledge. Compute Canada, which controls the construction of and access to computer resources by Canadian academics, and the High-Performance Computing Program of the State of New York have arisen as government-sponsored organizations for high-performance computing.

- The Chinese National Center for High-Performance Computing;
- The European High-Performance Computing Technology Platform.

Bioinformatics requires high-performance computers, which is why firms like Amazon and Microsoft have begun to offer these services. Moreover, the emergence of community computing has revolutionized how individuals connect in the field of bioinformatics. BOINC, a platform for cooperation that allows people to make their computers accessible for distributed computations for various projects, is an example of this. BOINC enables specialists to submit computing jobs, while non-experts, scientific enthusiasts, and/or volunteers can participate by devoting their computer resources to BOINC initiatives. Multiple biological scientific projects, like protein-ligand docking, simulations of malaria, and protein folding, are now accessible via BOINC.

2.6 2010–TODAY: PRESENT AND FUTURE PERSPECTIVES

Clearly Defining the Bioinformatician Profession

The rise of professional researchers, or bioinformaticians, is a new development in the discipline of bioinformatics. Even after more than

50 years in the field, “bioinformatician” is not a well-recognized term. According to some authors, the name “bioinformatician” should be reserved for individuals who specialize in the subject, such as those who build, manage, and utilize bioinformatics tools. On the other hand, it was proposed that the word “bioinformatician” be used for all those who utilize bioinformatics technology. Even humorous was the attempt to explain what a bioinformatician is not and how to avoid becoming one.

It is known that helpful communities such as SEQanswers and BioStar have grown substantially, as have user-friendly tools, which are frequently available through integrative Web servers such as Galaxy. Bioinformaticians are also in great demand in the government, business, and academic sectors. Colleges were entrusted with modifying their biological sciences programs to meet this criterion.

Now, life scientists who are not directly involved in a bioinformatics study must understand the complexity of the tools, refrain from misusing them, and accurately interpret the results.

The International Society for Computational Biology established criteria and requirements for the core abilities of a bioinformatician based on three user types (bioinformatics user, bioinformatics scientist, and bioinformatics engineer). It is crucial to possess “general biology knowledge, in-depth knowledge of at least one area of biology, and comprehension of biological data generation technologies,” as well as “current techniques, skills, and tools required for computational biology practice,” “[applying] statistical research methods in the contexts of molecular biology, genomics, medical, and population genetics research,” and “[applying] statistical research methods in the contexts of computation.”

Additional competencies were specified for the latter two groups. For example, the bioinformatics engineer was expected to “[apply] mathematical foundations, algorithmic principles, and computer science theory in the modeling and design of computer-based systems in a way that demonstrates comprehension of the tradeoffs involved in design choices,” while the bioinformatics scientist was expected to “[analyze] a problem and identify and define the computing requirements appropriate to its solution” (Gauthier, 2019).

Is the Term ‘Bioinformatics’ Now Obsolete?

Before attempting to characterize the bioinformatician profession, maybe the term “bioinformatics” should be defined. The use of computers has expanded to the majority of the natural sciences (physics, chemistry, mathematics, cryptography, etc.), but oddly, only biology has a distinct title for this use of computers ('bioinformatics'). How did this come to be?

First, it has been thought for a long time that biology is at the intersection of "hard" and "soft" topics. Understanding the structure of macromolecules was also required for the application of computers in biology (namely, nucleic acids and proteins). Consequently, compared to other "difficult" sciences, such as physics and mathematics, biology was computerized later. This is unsurprising, given that the original computers were designed to solve physics-related mathematical problems. During World War II, the ENIAC (1943–1966), one of the first fully electronic computers, was utilized to construct the hydrogen bomb.

The interplay of these variables may explain why the relationship between biology and computers was initially unclear. This may be why the word "bioinformatics" is still often used. One may dispute the continuous use of the phrase in the present period, considering that almost all research endeavors entail the use of a computer. Titus Brown, a bioinformatician, made an important comment in this respect during the 15th annual Bioinformatics Open-Source Conference. He provided a history of present bioinformatics from the perspective of a biologist in 2039. It is hard to differentiate Brown's prospective future from biology and bioinformatics. Both are characterized by the term "biology."

Towards Modeling Life as a Whole: Systems Biology

Late in the 20th century, the use of computers in biology increased. In conjunction with ever-improving laboratory equipment, their utilization has enabled increasingly sophisticated research activities. In the past, a doctorate dissertation may have focused on the sequencing of a single protein or gene, but Ph.D. students these days have the option to explore the collective genome of several microbial communities. Identifying the whole proteome of a sample is now feasible, whereas previously, it was difficult to pinpoint the fundamental structure of a protein. Even while various macromolecular categories (such as genomes, proteomics, and glycomics) have limited cross-pollination, biology has recently adopted a holistic approach.

In contrast to analyzing full genomes, transcriptomes, or metabolomes individually, whole organisms and their habitats will be modeled computationally with all molecular categories considered concurrently. Since all the genes, products, and known metabolic connections of *Mycoplasma genitalium* have been recreated *in silico*, it has been able to accomplish this accomplishment using a comprehensive cell model of the bacterium. Maybe soon we will get to see a full pluricellular model *in silico*. Even though simulating millions to trillions of cells may seem difficult, consider that we are already performing scientific accomplishments that were considered computationally or technically unachievable just five years ago.

CHAPTER 3

INTEGRAL COMPONENT OF BIOINFORMATICS

CONTENTS

3.1 INTRODUCTION

Bioinformatics, a rapidly growing science, brings biologists, computer scientists, and mathematicians together. The field known as "bioinformatics" would be formally defined in 1968. Bioinformatics is also referred to as computational biology. In the end, most computational biology labor is spent simulating biological systems. Bioinformatics is founded on two fundamental principles: the creation of novel software and algorithms and the analysis and interpretation of biological data utilizing such tools and algorithms (Tomita, M., 2012).

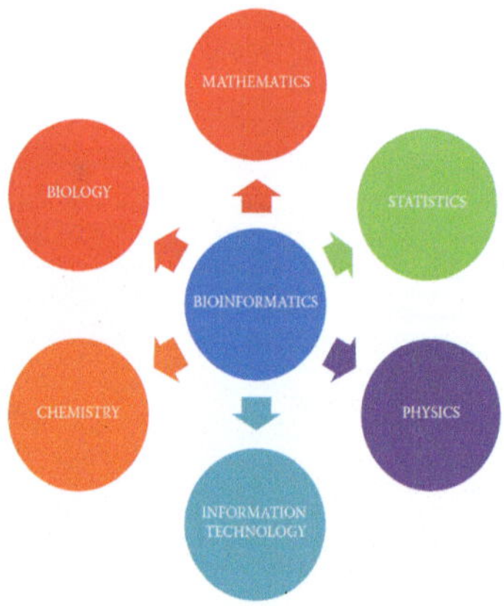

Figure 3.1: Bioinformatics: An inter-disciplinary area.

Source: Bioinformatics and RNA: A Practice-Based Approach - Scientific Figure on ResearchGate. Available from: https://www.researchgate.net/figure/Bioinformatics-An-Inter-disciplinary-Area_fig1_352196839 [accessed 25 Nov 2022]

Oxford Dictionaries define bioinformatics as "the collecting, processing, systematic analysis, and storage of biological data." This criterion indicates that even for a small life science organization, developing a single bioinformatics solution is a difficult task. This is especially true when one considers the immensity of data, its exponential growth, the intricacies of biological data sets, and the wide range of data types. As time passes, it becomes evident that no single answer will tackle all of the problems in bioinformatics. A growing school of thought holds that if bioinformatics aims to "enable the integration of biological data with knowledge resources from other disciplines," we must pursue an integrated strategy that uses existing solutions whenever possible. Furthermore, with the introduction of a new computer architecture known as web services, a technical platform capable of integrating and making available biological data has arisen.

Rapid sequencing of vast genomic areas is now achievable because of advances in molecular biology. Data-intensive projects such as the Human Genome Project highlight the importance of appropriately storing, classifying, and indexing sequence data. As a result, various sequence databases, such as GenBank and EMBL, have arisen. This study investigates the possible efficiency improvements that might arise from researchers working together, exchanging data, and using a holistic bioinformatics approach.

Because of the fast advancement of next-generation sequencing (NGS) technology and the concomitant growth in the volume of biological data, various data sources have been established to improve data administration, accessibility, and analysis. Data discovery, analysis, and retrieval from several data sources are becoming increasingly crucial in bioinformatics research. For each bioinformatics project, researchers must be able to rapidly query several data sources and then use the results for additional data analysis and keyword searches. Before the analyzed result can be comprehended and merged with data from a third data source, the data must be received from one data source, reformatted, and transferred to a second data source for analysis, for example. Massive volumes of current NGS data and other data types complicate and lengthen the data integration procedure. (Tomita, M. 2012)

3.2. COMPUTATIONAL BIOLOGY

The goal of computational biology is to learn and apply models of biological systems based on experimental data. These models could help answer questions like which nucleic acid or peptide sequences are responsible for which biological functions, which gene(s) cause which phenotype or behavior when expressed, which combination of changes in gene or protein expression or localization leads to which disease, and how changes in cellular organization influence cellular behavior. Even though the term "bioinformatics" is not often used, some scientists do.

The name for computer science in German is "Informatik," whereas the word for computational biology in German is "bioinformatik." The fact that one of the most prestigious publications in computational biology is called "Bioinformatics" adds to the misunderstanding. Others contend that bioinformatics focuses on the open interchange of biological data. Data from "bioinformatics" systems are commonly utilized for model creation by "computational biology" systems, and model outputs are routinely given back to "bioinformatics" databases for long-term storage. (Stegle, O. 2016).

Because it tries to construct models for a wide range of experimental data (including concentrations, sequences, and images) and biological systems, computational biology spans a broad field of research (such as molecules, cells, tissues, and organs). Furthermore, it employs various computational and mathematical approaches (e.g., complexity theory, algorithmics, machine learning, robotics, etc.).

Computer biologists' primary goal is to model biological issues as computational activities. This might mean adopting a unique approach to biological systems, questioning the traditional understanding of how system pieces are related, or synthesizing information from several sources into a more comprehensive model than previously tried. While acquiring a better understanding of the system is always worthwhile, it is crucial to remember that even relatively simple biological systems might be too complex for scientists to comprehend or predict their behavior fully. As a result, the ultimate aim may be the development of a model; the model should account for the most recent available experimental data. It has not been verified even if the model correctly predicts one or more future trials. Except under exceptional circumstances, a model may only be abandoned in favor of a superior one incorporating fresh discoveries.

Machine learning is fundamental to this strategy for generating models. Most modern machine learning applications begin by using statistical and computational approaches to generate models from vast existing datasets and then utilize these models to handle incoming data. Examples include:

- Learning to recognize human speech.
- Unlocking a mobile device with a fingerprint.
- Recognizing and categorizing spam emails.

Many machine learning applications continue to learn long after their initial training. They can either wait for more data to become available or pick which new data to utilize for training. Active machine learning is likely to have a significant impact on biomedical research in the future years (Stegle, O. 2016)

3.3. GENOMICS

The study of all or a portion of genetic or epigenetic sequence information of an organism to deduce the structure and function of the following biological products is called "genomics." The study of the interaction between a person's genetic composition and the biological processes, therapeutic interventions, and environmental variables that contribute to the development of sickness is known as genetics in medicine (Hartwell, 2011).

Many aspects of genomics other than individual genomes are critical to human health. Many other species genomes, including plants, insects, and viruses, interact with the human genome. Genomic research is considered to impact the health of all species, making it a priority. We supply genetic data and technologies that use what we have discovered about the human genome.

Genes and genomes are distinct disciplines of research. Genetics looks at DNA while investigating heredity, whereas genomics looks at DNA, its functions, and the technology that studies it. The genomic study examines genes of an organism and their interconnections to understand how they interact for the growth and development of the organism. In contrast, genetics analyzes the structure and function of a single gene.

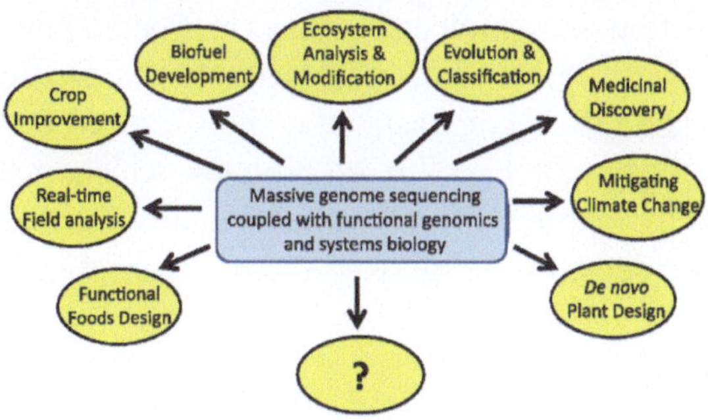

Figure 3.2: Genome sequencing and functional genomics: where do we go from here? Flow chart showing some of the current and future applications of functional genomics and NextGen genome/RNA sequencing.

Source: Mittler, R., & Shulaev, V. (2013). Functional genomics, challenges and perspectives for the future. Physiologia Plantarum, 148 3, 317-321.

Human genomics research and related biotechnologies have the potential to contribute to a variety of public health objectives, such as the reduction of global health disparities, by providing developing countries with reliable, effective, and cost-effective means of preventing, diagnosing, and treating the most prevalent diseases affecting their populations.

Given how quickly genomics is evolving as a science, the long-term influence on medical care is a vast unknown. It may. However, one day it will lead to better treatment and prevention strategies for a broad spectrum of incurable diseases. As a result, people must prepare for the challenges that this new field will bring, that the benefits are distributed fairly across all countries and that traditional, more established medical research and practice methods are not abandoned in favor of the novel possibilities offered by genomics. Even though most novel treatment options are often available in wealthier countries, low- and middle-income countries bear a disproportionate share of the global burden of illness and its effects. As a result of global health inequity, low and middle-income nations are handicapped in their pursuit of genetic research developments. Various reasons contribute to rising disparities in the global distribution of genetic technology, genomic research, and genomic service supply. One is a lack of necessary resources, such as health care facilities and services, or severe health issues, such as TB and HIV/AIDS (Hartwell, 2011).

3.4. PROTEOMICS

The critical function that molecules play in maintaining life has been recognized from the beginning of biological studies. Berzelius coined the name "protein" in 1838 to emphasize the significance of these molecules. Protein is derived from the Greek word proteios, which means "excellent." The proteome is the number of cell proteins at any moment.Proteomics is critical for disease detection, diagnosis, and monitoring.

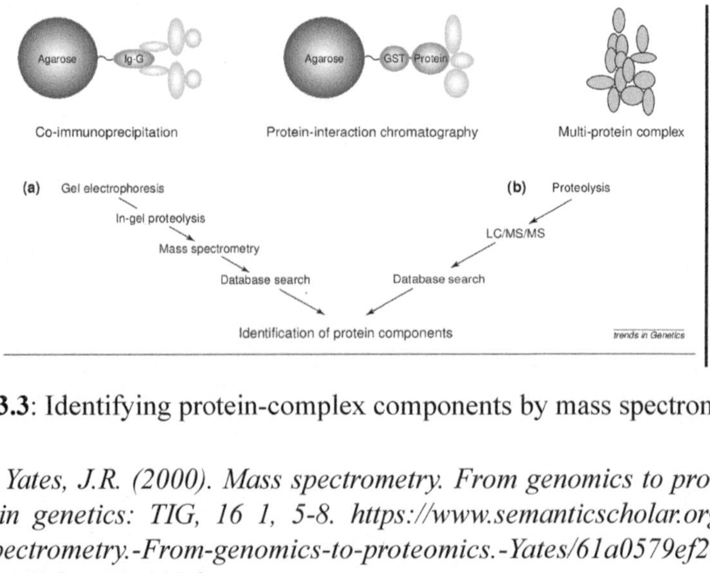

Figure 3.3: Identifying protein-complex components by mass spectrometry.

Source: Yates, J.R. (2000). Mass spectrometry. From genomics to proteomics. Trends in genetics: TIG, 16 1, 5-8. https://www.semanticscholar.org/paper/Mass-spectrometry.-From-genomics-to-proteomics.-Yates/61a0579ef24cc54ee5368d7e763dccc78a207dec

It is determined by variables such as their location, interactions, post-translational modifications, and rate of turnover. Marc Wilkins defined the "Protein Complement of a Genome" with the term "proteomics" in 1996. The proteome reveals the function of a majority of genes. The proteome of eukaryotic cells is dynamic and highly complex. Furthermore, proteins generated by bacteria are responsible for harmful activities; however, measuring these proteins is difficult due to the wide range of their characteristics. These characteristics include a variable amount, molecular size, hydrophobicity, and hydrophilicity.

Furthermore, it contributes to identifying new drugs by giving molecules to be used as targets. Proteomics investigates protein expression, structure, interactions, and alterations during various stages of development—the proteome changes over time, from cell to cell, and in response to environmental signals. Post-translational changes, which can occur in many locations and via various methods, add to the complexity of proteomics in eukaryotic cells. (Rasool, M. H. 2017). Proteomics is one of the most important ways to understand how genes operate while being significantly more complex than genomics. Analyzing the transcriptome or proteome, which can show changes in gene expression, can help differentiate between two biological states of the cell—using microarray chips to undertake broad transcriptome research. Microarrays, however, cannot immediately detect an increase in mRNA production. The amount of a particular protein is regulated to a considerable extent by the translational regulation and control systems of the host and the amount of its matching messenger RNA. As a result, proteomics is regarded as the gold standard for characterizing living entities. Proteins may be isolated and purified using various chromatographic methods, including affinity chromatography, size exclusion chromatography, and ion exchange chromatography. The Western blotting technique and the enzyme-linked immunosorbent test are two methods for examining proteins (ELISA). These methodologies are insensitive to measuring protein expression levels and can only analyze several proteins. To separate complicated protein samples, two-dimensional gel electrophoresis, two-dimensional differential gel electrophoresis, and SDS-PAGE are all utilized (2D-DIGE).

3.5. PHARMACOGENOMICS

The study of how genetics interacts with pharmacological responses is known as pharmacogenomics. In the long term, it should assist doctors in prescribing the appropriate drugs in the appropriate dosages for each unique patient. It is a type of customized medicine in which therapies are tailored to specific needs of each patient.

Our genetic make-up affects sensitivity to drugs in the same way it determines the color of our hair and eyes. Genes supply the necessary DNA instructions for the production of specific proteins. In various animals, the same gene has many variants. Minor differences exist in DNA sequences in variants. There are both familiar and unusual varieties. Some, such as disease-linked gene variants, significantly impact health.

Specific proteins are now known to impair the efficiency of numerous medicines. Pharmacogenomics is the study of these proteins and the differences in their coding genes. Drug-modifying enzymes discovered in the liver belong to this class of proteins. Physiological factors can affect drug potency. The genes that code for these liver enzymes have a lot of opportunity for genetic variation, and even little alterations can significantly influence the safety or efficacy of a medicine (Rasool, M. H. 2017).

About 25% of all drugs are thought to interact with the CYP2D6 enzyme present in the liver. Take the pain medication codeine as an example; it may be converted into even more potent morphine. About 160 variants may be detected in the CYP2D6 gene. The DNA sequences of a couple of persons are slightly wrong. There are those whose appearance has been drastically changed. Most of these variances have little effect on how people react to the medicine.

This is because each cell contains identical duplicates of all its genes. Rarely may a person have hundreds or thousands of working copies of CYP2D6. More drug-degrading enzyme CYP2D6 is generated in persons with many copies of the gene. Due to the excellent efficiency with which their bodies metabolize codeine into morphine, a usual dose may be too much for them. Some CYP2D6 genotypes, however, produce a less effective enzyme. Because of these changes, codeine is digested slowly or not at all, diminishing or eliminating its analgesic effects. Their physicians may recommend they try something different to aid them.

Age, weight, gender, liver function, and renal function are only some aspects that are being taken into account while prescribing drugs. Several frequently prescribed drugs have been revealed to have gene changes that alter patient reactions. In such a situation, doctors might be able to modify patients' treatment programs down to the specific dose.

It could be beneficial in illness diagnosis to discover how a patient responds to various medications. (Rasool, 2017).

3.6. PHARMACOGENETICS

The study of how the genetic make-up of a person impacts how effectively a medicine works in their body is referred to as "pharmacogenomics." Pharmaceutical genomics integrates the analysis of genes and their activities with pharmaceutical technology to develop safe and effective medications that may be supplied in several ways based on the genetic profile of the particular patient.

Although the effectiveness of various treatments varies widely, many are marketed as though they are uniformly beneficial. It can be challenging to determine who will respond well to a therapy, who will not respond, and who will have harmful side effects (called adverse drug reactions). Unwanted pharmaceutical responses are responsible for a significantly growing healthcare costs and accompanying human misery in the United States (Berrettini, 2014). Scientists are attempting to determine whether and how different forms of genetic diversity impact the response of the body to certain medications. These DNA differences will affect how well a treatment works and the likelihood of undesirable side effects in a patient. Some diseases that alter the reaction of a person to medicine include clopidogrel resistance, warfarin sensitivity, warfarin resistance, malignant hyperthermia, Stevens-Johnson syndrome/toxic epidermal necrolysis, and thiopurine S-methyltransferase deficiency.

Because pharmacogenomics is still in its infancy, clinical researchers always search for innovative strategies. Pharmacogenomics will provide personalized medicines for disorders such as asthma, Alzheimer's, cancer, and cardiovascular disease.

Pharmacogenomics is a critical component of precision medicine for tailoring treatment to an individual or group of patients. Pharmacogenomics is a discipline of medicine that studies the influence of genes on how people react to drugs. People genetic make-up determines the outcome of treatment. Pharmacogenomics can help the individual to assess if a treatment is likely to be helpful and safe for the individual to consume, which can improve his/her health.

3.7. CHEMINFORMATICS

Computers and databases are utilized in cheminformatics to acquire insight into chemical challenges, such as the *in silico* mapping of chemical space. This is a fictitious zone containing all potential chemicals and compounds.

Approaches based on cheminformatics are beneficial in drug development and other sectors where many chemicals must be examined for a limited range of attributes.

Cheminformatics is an information technology branch focusing on gathering, storing, analyzing, and altering chemical data. The most prevalent sorts of chemical data of interest include formulae, structures, characteristics, spectra, and activities of tiny molecules (biological or industrial). Originally intended to aid in the discovery and development of medicines, chemoinformatics has since found various uses in biology, chemistry, and biochemistry.

Hit enrichment curves are frequently used in virtual drug development screening to assess the performance of ranking algorithms based on their capacity to detect early enrichment. Unfortunately, when comparing competing algorithms' performance, researchers seldom consider the inherent uncertainty in forecasting such curves. Because researchers prefer to focus on small testing fractions, uncertainty is prevalent. Correlation between competing algorithms and correlation between distinct testing fractions within a single algorithm are two examples of a correlation that are frequently neglected yet can substantially impede correct inference. Furthermore, researchers prefer to study data across the whole curve rather than focusing on a small number of testing fractions. Those interested in both the entire curve and a portion of the testing fractions can profit from the inferential procedures given in the study. After comparing it to four other techniques of doing such tests and calculating (pointwise) confidence intervals, a newly developed EmProc methodology is demonstrated to be the most successful for hypothesis testing. It is advised to utilize confidence bands based on EmProc for the whole-curve inference that is both comprehensive and narrow. Although the hit enrichment curve is the focus of this article, lift curves are also significant owing to their extensive application in machine learning and should not be disregarded. The authors' inference methods are likewise questionable when applied to enrichment factors. (Berrettini, W. H. 2014).

3.8. STRUCTURAL GENOMICS OR STRUCTURAL BIOINFORMATICS

Structural genomics aims to visualize the three-dimensional structure of every protein using either experimental, computational, or a combination of these methods. Problem-solving and hypothesis-testing research led to the discovery of the first 3-D protein structures. The structure-determination process is critical because it discloses previously unknown features of biological processes, such as molecular recognition, enzyme activity, and energy transfer. The discovery of new links between amino acid sequences and protein structures has been the most significant advance in structural biology. To understand more about proteins' complicated 3-D structure, we need to create new computational tools for concepts like fold, protein family, and superfamily. Identifying the whole protein repertoire of an organism, producing high-resolution physical and genetic maps, and sequencing the genome are all genomic approaches.

Both shotgun sequencing and clone-by-clone sequencing are employed to finish the genome sequence. To begin, the fragments are cloned-by-clone aligned into contigs. Following that, plasmid and cosmid clones are created by connecting the separate parts. The individual clones that comprise the contig are then sequenced. Shotgun sequencing can investigate every clone in a genomic library since it requires several rounds of sequencing. The gathered nucleotide sequence data is assembled using assembler software into a genomic sequence.

Structural genomics (SG) aims to publish the three-dimensional structures of all physiologically significant macromolecules, with proteins as the primary focus. At the turn of the century, several SG consortia were created in the Americas, Europe, and Asia.

Naturally, there is no way to compare the number of known protein structures to the number of genetic sequences. Unlike sequences with a virtually limitless number of alternative outcomes, the "fold space" is finite. There is no reason to expect that the nearly 10,000 protein sequence families discovered thus far would "explode." The SG intends to have one representative structure available for each protein family. To get there, SG laboratories have established techniques for high-throughput target selection, protein expression and purification, crystallization, X-ray crystallography, and nuclear magnetic resonance structure analysis. Existing genetic data must guide the selection of proteins for structural determination within SG programs. Common structural analogies are thus avoided in favor of structural uniqueness.

3.9. COMPARATIVE GENOMICS

Comparative genomics is a branch of biology that studies the similarities and differences between the complete genome sequences of different species.

Researchers can identify areas of resemblance and dissimilarity by carefully investigating the traits that distinguish various organisms.

The first step in studying the genome is to discover DNA sequences that have been "conserved," or retained, in different species across millions of years. It looks for life-sustaining genes and the genetic signals that regulate their expression across species. This advances our understanding of the interactions between genes and other biological processes, which may lead to innovative methods for illness prevention and treatment in the future.

Furthermore, understanding evolution using comparative genomes is a practical approach. Scientists can better understand how the appearance, behavior, and biology of living things have evolved by exploiting and analyzing evolutionary links between species and the consequent changes in their DNA.

Comparative genomics is used in agriculture, biotechnology, and zoology to learn about the frequently minute distinctions between animal species as DNA sequencing technology advances and costs fall. These activities have contributed to improved living conditions for domesticated animals, new insights into particular evolutionary routes, and novel conservation measures for at-risk species.

DNA (deoxyribonucleic acid) is a molecular chain that makes up most known living beings' genomes. It contains the genes that code for proteins and the regulatory sequences that control the expression of those genes. The arrangement of the four building blocks of DNA—adenine (A), thymine (T), cytosine (C), and guanine (G)—along the double helix determines the protein the gene produces. Using comparative genomics has resulted in several fundamental discoveries. Comparative genomics research is frequently used to answer fundamental concerns regarding human evolution, behavior, metabolism, and disease susceptibility. We are learning about previously undiscovered links and similarities across species at the genetic, behavioral, neurological, and developmental levels as a result of these investigations. Some scholars are using comparative genomics to discover the chromosomal underpinnings of disease in animals to understand the origins of human diseases better (Berrettini, W. H. 2014).

3.10. BIOPHYSICS

Biophysics has made it possible to comprehend the mechanics of biomolecules, the movement and function of diverse cell components, and the operation of the brain, circulatory, and immune systems. Specialists from mathematics, chemistry, physics, engineering, pharmacology, and materials science collaborate in the expanding scientific discipline of biophysics to examine and create novel techniques for understanding the workings of biology or life in general.

Physicists employ mathematical models to comprehend their surroundings better. 'It is all about figuring out how living things function for life scientists. These systems are highly complex, ranging from molecules and cells to living beings and whole ecosystems. Experiments in biology in the twenty-first century generate massive volumes of data. How could researchers interpret this data and speculate on the underlying mechanics of these systems?

Biophysicists can help in this situation. Biophysicists can investigate a wide range of biological questions due to their extensive training in the quantitative sciences of physics, mathematics, and chemistry, including how nerve cells communicate, how plant cells convert light into energy, how changes in the DNA of healthy cells can cause them to transform into cancer cells, and many more.

Biophysicists are interested in a wide range of scientific challenges, such as those concerning sickness, hunger, energy, and technology. Finally, biophysicists play an essential role in developing solutions to significant challenges that humankind faces today and in the future.

In 1953, scientists first realized that biophysics could be used to derive the structure of DNA; this discovery was critical in our understanding the significance of DNA as a life-sustaining blueprint.

Thousands of DNA sequences from humans and other animals are now accessible for examination. These huge data sets are analyzed using biophysical techniques.

Biophysicists create and apply computational modeling tools to study and manipulate the three-dimensional shapes and structures of proteins, viruses, and other complex molecules; this knowledge is critical for identifying new therapeutic targets and understanding of the role proteins play in tumor progression.

Biophysicists research cellular signaling and hormone transfer. Biophysicists used fluorescent tags to make cells shine like fireflies under the microscope to investigate the intricate intracellular transport system. Neural networks are computer models developed by biophysicists to mimic the functioning of the brain and nervous system. These discoveries provide information on how the brain perceives and processes sight and sound (Berrettini, W. H. 2014).

3.11 BIOMEDICAL INFORMATICS/ MEDICAL INFORMATICS

Biomedical informatics is a branch of health informatics that uses data to aid physicians, researchers, and scientists in promoting and delivering healthcare. Biomedicine has given rise to biomedical informatics, which uses natural scientific principles, most notably biology and biochemistry, to treat patients and provide healthcare. However, as the biotechnology sector has evolved and personal health data has been more digitalized, biomedical informatics has become more reliant on software, artificial intelligence, and cloud computing.

Biomedical informatics connects medical disciplines, provides clinical insights, identifies sickness, treatment, and response patterns, and offers new avenues for scientific and medical research. This is accomplished by combining traditional scientific studies with massive data sets and novel information presentation methods.

Cloud computing has enabled significant advances in DNA sequencing and genomics. Advanced medical imaging and visualization technologies, such as 3-D printing and ultra-high resolution screens, provide clinicians and researchers with access to many low-cost, high-quality data sources.

Biomedical informatics may help in various fields of medical research and treatment. Roger Day, a researcher at the University of Pittsburgh, Department of Biomedical Informatics, has investigated how computational and biomathematical modeling tools might lead to deeper biological information that can tailor cancer treatment to individual patients.

Furthermore, biomedical informaticians in the pharmaceutical industry design and operate pharmacovigilance systems to improve the safety of clinical trials and drug testing. Pharmacovigilance systems use data science and predictive analytics to detect problems in drug trials and unreported adverse effects. Biomedical informatics is concerned with genomics, proteomics (the comprehensive study of proteins), pharmacology, and other medical challenges. Furthermore, it demonstrates the use of traditional and computational methodologies in biology and medicine.

3.12 MATHEMATICAL BIOLOGY

Mathematicians and biologists have a long history of fruitful collaboration, especially in medicine. Mathematical innovations have been used and developed in the life sciences. Examples include the development of stochastic processes and statistical techniques to address various population issues in demography, ecology, genetics, and epidemics. Most biologists', physicists,' chemists,' and engineers' work involves synthesizing and analyzing mathematical structures. Key mathematical developments and applications influenced by biological sciences are related to Pythagoras, Aristotle, Fibonacci, Cardano, Bernoulli, Euler, Fourier, Laplace, Gauss, von Helmholtz, Riemann, Einstein, Thompson, Turing, Wiener, von Neumann, Thom, and Keller.

Despite encompassing all fields of mathematics, mathematical biology is a vastly diverse field that defies categorization into standard mathematical inquiry categories (real and complex analysis, integral and differential systems, metamathematics, algebra, geometry, number theory, topology, probability and statistics, and computer sciences) (real and complex analysis, integral and differential systems, metamathematics, algebra, geometry, number theory, topology, probability, and statistics, as well as computer sciences). The field combines fundamental mathematics with biological problems. The importance of mathematics in biology stems partly from the use of statistics and calculus to quantify phenomena in the life sciences but also from the sophisticated perspective that data organization and the recognition and analysis of emergent structures can bring to complex real-world systems. Mathematicians, physicists, chemists, engineers, and physicians devised and used mathematical methodologies in biological research. It isn't easy to comprehend mathematics' enormous impact on biology.

There are important issues that require mathematical research in almost every aspect of life and medical sciences. They are not standard mathematical problems, but they can combine new mathematical structures and provide new perspectives on well-known ones. For example, Rene Thom used topology and singularity theory to study developmental biology. He established and investigated conventional mathematical models that reflected the most significant components of developmental events to understand the underlying biological processes better. Pattern formation in nature research, which began with the work of D'Arcy Thompson and led to the creation of acceptable mathematical models for reaction-diffusion systems, continues to contribute to the study of a wide range of fields today. Furthermore, stochastic process techniques have been developed and used for many biological problems, including population genetics and molecular biology. Numerous more complex mathematical discoveries have aided the study of biology.

3.13. COMPUTATIONAL CHEMISTRY

Because of computational chemistry, the emergence of enantioselectivity in transition metal-catalyzed asymmetric synthesis may be understood mechanistically. Numerous chemical processes, including hydrogenation catalyzed by rhodium, dihydroxylation catalyzed by osmium, alkylation catalyzed by zinc, cyclopropanation catalyzed by copper, and sulfoxidation catalyzed by vanadium, have profited from calculations.

Asymmetric synthesis is still difficult to grasp conceptually. To begin, the computational technique must be capable of simulating energy changes typically less than 3 kcal / mol. Because of the fault cancellation that occurs when comparing relative paths leading to R and S products, this is often handled utilizing contemporary QM or QM/MM approaches and increasing computational power. On the other hand, the molecular intricacy of the processes involved in asymmetric catalysis has become a barrier to broader, practical black-box application of computational chemistry to asymmetric synthesis. Because asymmetric catalysis is challenging to achieve, the systems in which it occurs are typically complex.

Computational chemistry has played an essential role in understanding mechanical complexity thus far because it can learn about intermediates that are difficult to identify experimentally owing to kinetics. It is critical to emphasize that computations often follow the experiment, validating previous knowledge and providing an advantage. Determining the origins of enantioselectivity is an excellent place to start when developing new systems that may overcome the limitations of existing systems and, therefore, be effective for process optimization.

Future scientific breakthroughs must focus on utilizing computational chemistry's ability for efficient prediction to build brand-new approaches from the ground up, ultimately revolutionizing drug discovery, materials science, and environmental sustainability. Rather than developing new techniques for measuring energy, which appear to be adequate, the plan for achieving this goal comprises increasing the use of computers for tedious tasks such as conformation searches and deep investigation of complex mechanical landscapes. Many jobs have always required human labor because developing complex systems would take too long. If these minor improvements can be made, the prospect for a significant increase in computer studies of enantioselective synthesis, which may become an essential field of practical application for computational chemistry, is quite promising. (Berrettini, W. H. 2014).

3.14. FUNCTIONAL GENOMICS

The study of "functional genomics" is concerned with the role that genes and intergenic areas play in diverse biological processes. Scientists in this subject routinely do "genome-wide" analysis (i.e., on all or some genes/regions at once) to restrict the pool of candidate genes/locations for future investigation.

Functional genomics aims to understand the intricate interplay between genes, proteins, and other elements of a live organism that leads to a specific phenotype. Available genomics studies the dynamic expression of gene products under particular situations, such as in response to a disease or throughout development. Functional genomics aims to use what we know about how genes work to create a model that establishes a link between genotype and phenotype.

Transcriptomics, proteomics, and metabolomics characterize the transcripts, proteins, and metabolites that comprise a biological system, and their integration is intended to offer a comprehensive description of the system.

Functional genomics, a subset of genomics, seeks to establish whether there is a link between genetic composition and observable behaviors. The objective is to understand how genes work and interact with one another. RNA interference (RNAi), mutagenesis, mass spectrometry, genome annotation, and other methods are commonly used to explore gene and protein function. Most functional genomics research uses model species of plants, animals, and humans since it is straightforward and affordable to monitor gene inheritance through several generations of studied organisms. Comparative genomics approaches may be used to better comprehend larger genomes by expanding on what has been learned from model species.

Because of advancements in functional genomics, high-throughput approaches for expression profiling in various parts of the brain and cell types have been created. When cutting-edge technologies are integrated with well-planned studies and tested using recognized molecular and cellular-based approaches to develop a new paradigm, the pathophysiological pathways underlying Parkinson's disease may be studied. Some genes and transcript sets comprising various signaling pathways can be examined *in vitro* in the midbrain, SNPC, and striatum of relevant Parkinson's disease animal models and the brains of postmortem Parkinson's disease patients.

3.15. PHARMACOINFORMATICS

Since the 1990s, the third-generation cephalosporin ceftazidime has been in widespread use. This is frequently used to treat infections, even the most severe and resistant forms. Ceftazidime-averbatan was authorized by the US Food and Drug Administration in 2015 to treat complex urinary tract infections and severe abdominal infections when coupled with metronidazole. Because of its high blood concentration, low protein binding rate, renal clearance, extensive *in vivo* distribution, and blood-brain barrier penetration, CAZ is ideally suited for intramuscular or intravenous administration. As predicted, CAZ harms various body organs, including the central nervous, circulatory, urinary, and gastrointestinal systems. Drug toxicity has two effects: the detrimental effects of the medication itself and the possible hazards provided by contaminants in the drug production process. The discovery and control of impurities in medicines, particularly the management of genetic toxicity contaminants, is mandated by several nations' and international organizations' drug regulatory agencies. However, there has been little investigation into the risks of CAZ pollutants.

The structural features of impurities cannot be separated from their toxicity. Computers have been widely used to forecast toxicity based on structure-activity connections in Europe and the United States. Recent research has investigated the link between cephalosporin structure and toxicity using molecular docking, computational chemistry, and the zebrafish embryo toxicity test. The C-3 and C-7 side chains are principally responsible for cephalosporins' and their impurities' teratogenic, neurotoxic, and cardiotoxic actions.

The pkCSM ADMET descriptors algorithm protocol1 and the Discover Studio 4.0 application were used to identify drug pharmacokinetic (PK) features. The 2D polar surface area and lipophilicity levels as atom-based LogP are primary chemical descriptors strongly linked with PK characteristics. Different variables influence the rate and degree of drug absorption, including skin permeability, intestinal absorption, and the presence of a P-glycoprotein substrate or inhibitor. Factors such as blood-brain barrier permeability, central nervous system permeability, and distribution volume all impact drug distribution. Metabolic predictions are made using CYP substrate and inhibitor models. The total clearance model and the renal OCT2 substrate are utilized to forecast excretion. The toxicology of a medicine can be predicted by using tests for AMES toxicity, hERG inhibition, hepatotoxicity, and skin sensitivity. We computed and examined how well these variables matched within their projected ranges.

3.16. IN SILICO ADME-TOX PREDICTION

To enhance pharmaceutical quality control, scholars applied in silico approaches to anticipate the pharmacokinetics of ceftazidime (CAZ) and its impurities (ADMET). We employed docking and quantitative structure-activity relationship tools Discovery Studio 4.0, OECD QSAR Toolbox 4.1, Toxtree, and the pkCSM approach to developing reliable predictions. Impurity A (2-CAZ) pharmacokinetics and toxicity were found to be equivalent to ceftazidime.

The biological effects of impurity B, commonly known as the CAZ E-isomer, differ from those of CAZ. As a result, scholars examined impurity B to see how it might influence the life of the drug. The pollutants D and I are particularly harmful due to their high lipophilicity, excellent intestine absorption, and poor elimination from the body. Impurity D is highly harmful to the nervous system and the genome. It is critical to keep the level of impurity D low. When impurity F is combined with the C-3 side chain of CAZ, a quaternary amine group is formed, which is more dangerous than either impurity alone.

The most hazardous functional groups of CAZ are the C-7 acetates, C-3 quaternary amines, and the beta-lactam ring in the nucleus. According to a certain study, CAZ includes neurotoxic contaminants B and D due to genetic contamination. This *in-silico* technique may assess the toxicity of impurities and other cephalosporins.

The structural features of impurities cannot be separated from their toxicity. SARs, or structure-activity relationships, have been widely employed for toxicity prediction in Europe and the United States. Recent research has investigated the link between cephalosporin structure and toxicity using molecular docking, computational chemistry, and the zebrafish embryo toxicity test. The C-3 and C-7 side chains are principally responsible for cephalosporins' and their impurities' teratogenic, neurotoxic, and cardiotoxic actions. This work aimed to explain the structure-toxicity correlations of cephalosporins thoroughly and to utilize software to evaluate the toxicity of ceftazidime impurities reported in the Europium Pharmacopoeia.

3.17. AGROINFORMATICS / AGRICULTURAL INFORMATICS

Legislators, extension workers, and farmers now have access to the tools they need to find digital solutions to the critical difficulties they face, thanks to data and technology. The FAO is better equipped to accomplish its strategic goals of encouraging sustainable agriculture and early warning systems when it has access to data that is more precise, integrated, and multidimensional. This is because it reveals new opportunities and improves the design of programs, as well as the monitoring of progress, the evaluation of repercussions, and the provision of services.

The AgroInformatics department of the FAO works at achieving a more seamless integration of cutting-edge information technology. In addition to this, it makes use of agroinformatics to promote the production and distribution of digital public goods, such as data and information that can be utilized in the food and agricultural industries in a variety of different contexts.

One of the most significant things that the Organization is able to achieve with information technology is the establishment, improvement, and expansion of digital public goods related to information and communications technologies and agroinformatics. The Food and Agriculture Organization of the United Nations (FAO) has the goal of ensuring that decisions are made based on facts, that natural resources are managed in a way that is both sustainable and efficient, that output is increased, and that early warning systems are enhanced. This is contingent on the interoperability of the geospatial data FAO as well as the cost-effective maintenance and long-term sustainability of the geospatial applications of FAO.

The study of agricultural data, how to process it, and how to put up agricultural data systems is what is known as the field of agro informatics. Agro informatics refers to the branch of agricultural study that makes use of computer technology and other cutting-edge research approaches. It is largely concerned with the organization, evaluation, and use of agricultural data by means of information technology.The integration of artificial intelligence, neural networks, decision support systems, geographic information systems, genetic algorithms, and programming languages is at the heart of agro informatics. This allows for the development of robust software that makes agriculture more accessible, predictable, and ready for the digital age.

A few current examples of the importance of agroinformatics include: food security, sustainable agriculture, bio-energy, environmental research, natural resource conservation, carbon accounting, combating global climate change, commodity trading, economic research, education, health research, policy formulation, and decision-making. Agro informatics, sometimes referred to as "e-agriculture," is a field of study that promotes the dissemination of technology, information, and agricultural services. As a result, it enables farmers to increase their income. In the last 10 years, a number of research and development programs have been started in order to leverage the potential of information and communication technology to increase agricultural efficiency, raise overall production, and advance sustainable development. Agroinformatics has established connections between agricultural systems, environmentally responsible development, and the implementation of innovative technological practices.

CHAPTER 4

TYPES OF BIOLOGICAL DATA?

CONTENTS

Biological data refers to any information that describes the biological, genetic, biochemical, and/or physiological characteristics, composition, or functions of the substances to be analyzed with the Goods. Biological data includes processed nucleotide sequence data, but instrument data does not.

4.1. GENOME SEQUENCE DATA.

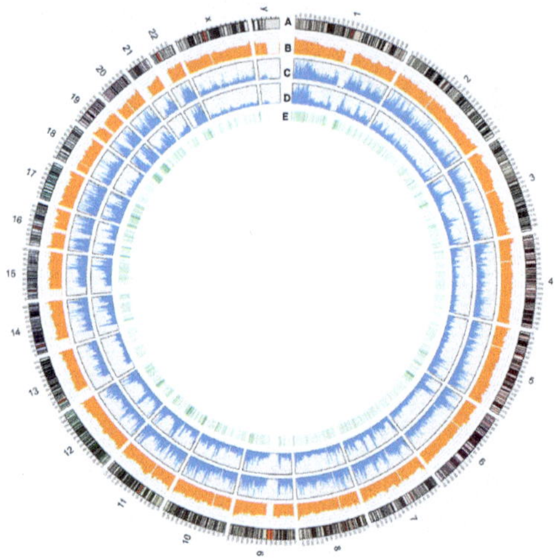

Figure 4.1: Graphic Representation of the Whole Genome of Two Single YH Cells (A) Karyotype of the human reference genome (Hg18). (B) GC content distribution of the reference genome (height of orange rectangles ranges from 0%-70%, bin = 1 Mb). (C) Whole-genome coverage of YH-2 (height of blue rectangles ranges from 03-403, bin = 1 Mb). (D) Whole-genome coverage of YH-1 (height of blue rectangles ranges from 03-403, bin = 1 Mb). (E) Gene density across the reference genome (Hg18) (gradually changing green represents from 0 to 30 genes per 100 kb). See also Figure S1.

Source: Single-Cell Exome Sequencing and Monoclonal Evolution of a JAK2-Negative Myeloproliferative Neoplasm - Scientific Figure on ResearchGate. Available from: https://www.researchgate.net/figure/Graphic-Representation-of-the-Whole-Genome-of-Two-Single-YH-Cells-A-Karyotype-of-the_fig1_221670048 [accessed 25 Nov 2022]

The Genome Sequence Data (GSD) database contains nucleotide sequences and biological and bibliographical information about them that are accessible to the public.

Researchers can use sophisticated computational and statistical techniques to decode the functional information encoded in DNA sequence thanks to genomic data sequence. These data science tools are utilized in genomic medicine to assist researchers and clinicians in comprehending the effects of genetic variations on human health and disease. (Trajanoski, Z. 2014).

In the 1990s, the field of genomic data was established to combine two laboratory procedures:

- Performing experiments to generate genomic data and analyse the genomes of living organisms.
- Data analysis: making predictions based on available genomic data using algorithms and software in addition to analyzing and visualizing genomic data using statistical and computational tools.

Each action contributes to the collection and analysis of vast quantities of genomic data.

How do scientists study and use genomic data?

Why Do Genomics Projects Require Such an Abundance of Data?

As a result of the Human Genome Project, the first sequence of the chemical bases (or "letters") — As, Cs, Gs, and Ts — in the human genome was successful, human genomics gained widespread attention in the early 2000s. Each of the trillions of cells that make up the human body contains the entire genome, or blueprint for our DNA. The majority of cells contain two copies of the genome, totaling about 6 billion DNA letters.

To gain a deeper understanding of how the genome affects human health and disease, scientists are producing more genomic data than ever before. These statistics were compiled by millions of individuals from a variety of populations around the globe. A single sequence of the human genome would require 200 gigabytes of storage space, roughly equivalent to 200 copies of Jaws. Globally generated genome-sequence data will require 40 exabytes of storage space by 2025. That is equivalent to nearly one billion DVDs of Jaws! In comparison, five exabytes would be sufficient to store every human word ever spoken.

To find and interpret the biological information buried within the DNA of each individual and to manage the massive amounts of data generated by genomics research projects, scientists need specialized computational and analysis tools. Researchers use aligners to pinpoint the location of specific DNA sequence fragments within each segment of a reference genome sequence (Trajanoski, Z. 2014).The "variant callers" then indicate where a particular human genome sequence differs from other human genome sequences. These genomic variations vary in size. Single-nucleotide polymorphisms, also known as structural variants, are chromosomal abnormalities that can range in size from a single DNA letter to a large number of DNA letters. These genomic variations may cause cancer, inherited rare disorders, or other more common diseases.z

How Do Scientists Manage and Store Such Vast Quantities of Genomic Data?

Using a variety of computer systems and applications, experts in both genomics and computer technology manage and store genomic data. As part of research networks, data analysis and coordination centers are increasingly providing these services.

Generating genomic data requires substantial financial support from organizations like the National Human Genome Research Institute (NHGRI), which annually contributes more than $125 million to genomic data science initiatives. Frequently, the generated data resources are made available to the broader scientific community to facilitate additional data analyses. They categorize and provide information regarding the human genome, including gene locations and DNA variants.

The National Institutes of Health (NIH) and its STRIDES project collaborate with numerous private and commercial clouds. These programs provide the necessary security and privacy safeguards for hosting genomic data as well as storage and computing infrastructure, with a focus on protecting human genomic data. (Trajanoski, Z. 2014).

What Are the Societal, Legal, and Ethical Implications of Sharing Genomic Information?

Because information about the genome sequence of a person is linked to complex privacy and identity issues, genomic research entails a set of ethical obligations.

- **Consent**. Before sequencing the genome of an individual, researchers typically obtain their informed consent. To obtain such informed consent, however, researchers must disclose how they intend to use and distribute the resulting genome-sequence data.

- **Confidentiality**. Robust computational tools can link de-identified genome sequence data to the individual whose DNA was sequenced under specific circumstances. These tools can be utilized for practical purposes, such as identifying criminals who left DNA at the scene of a crime. However, the societal benefits of using genomic data in this manner must outweigh the potential risks.
- **Artificial intelligence (AI)**: AI tools aid researchers in their search for hidden DNA patterns in vast amounts of genome sequence data. However, because AI algorithms frequently lack transparency, biases can enter DNA data undetected. Extensive ethics research will be required in this field to navigate the specific differences between the most recent AI methods and the more traditional genomic data science techniques (which rely on human intelligence for the interpretation of the results). AI methods have many potential benefits, but they also reach conclusions in ways that humans do not, necessitating a thorough examination of their ethical implications.

In light of these considerations, data scientists and genomics researchers must be cognizant of the repercussions of their work and collaborate closely with ethicists.

4.2. GENE VARIATION DATA

Genomic variation Data are differences in the DNA sequences of individuals or populations that are objectively observable. Some variants have no biological impact, while others have no impact on biological function (for example, a mutation that results in a genetic disease).

Understanding genomic variation in families and populations enables us to comprehend how our genetic make-up varies between individuals. It may help us to comprehend why members of the same family have varying blood types and eye colors. Genomic variation could also explain why certain populations or individuals within populations are more susceptible to particular diseases (Dunnen, J. T. 2011).

Genetic Variation Data Sources

'The DNA sequence of a gene can be altered in numerous ways. Gene variants, also known as mutations, can have a variety of effects on the health of an individual, depending on where they occur and whether they alter the function of specific proteins. Types of variants include the following:

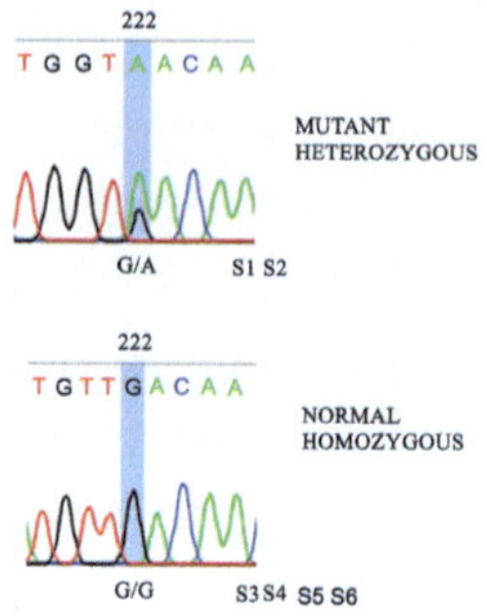

Figure 4.2: The pattern of the observed substitution mutation within the DNA chromatogram of the targeted 320 bp amplicons within the PROZ gene.

Source: The relation of PROZ1 polymorphism and risk of early fetal loss in the diagnosis of Iraqi patient with Antiphospholipid syndrome - Scientific Figure on ResearchGate. Available from: https://www.researchgate.net/figure/The-pattern-of-the-observed-substitution-mutation-within-the-DNA-chromatogram-of-the_fig3_346041615 [accessed 25 Nov 2022]

i. Substitution: This type of variation involves the substitution of one DNA nucleotide for another. Substitution variants can be further classified based on the effect they have on the production of proteins from the altered gene.

- Missense: A missense variant is a type of substitution in which a change in a nucleotide causes the protein produced by the gene to contain a different amino acid than was originally present. The amino acid change may affect the functionality of the protein.
- Nonsense: Another type of substitution is the nonsense variant. Instead of altering a single amino acid, the altered DNA sequence produces a premature stop signal that signals the cell to cease protein production. The shortened protein of this type of variant may not function, function improperly, or degrade.

ii. Insertion: The insertion of one or more nucleotides into a gene to alter its DNA sequence. Consequently, the function of the protein produced by the gene may be compromised.

iii. Deletion: A deletion modifies the DNA sequence of a gene by removing at least one nucleotide. Larger deletions can eliminate an entire gene or several nearby genes, whereas smaller deletions remove only one or a few nucleotides. The function of the protein or proteins affected by the DNA deletion may change.

iv. Deletion-Insertion: This variant arises when insertion and deletion simultaneously occur in the same region of the gene. A deletion-insertion variant is one in which at least one nucleotide is deleted and at least one is added. However, the modification must be substantial enough to distinguish it from a simple replacement. The function of the resulting protein may not be as intended. Both insertion-deletion and deletion-insertion refer to the same variant. (Dunnen, J. T. 2011).

v. Duplication: When a section of one or more nucleotides in a gene is duplicated and repeated next to the original DNA sequence, a duplication occurs. This kind of variation may alter the function of the protein encodedby the gene.

vi. Inversion: During an inversion, which modifies multiple nucleotides in a gene, the original sequence of nucleotides is exchanged for the same sequence in reverse order.

vii. Frameshift: A reading frame consists of three nucleotide groups, each of which corresponds to an amino acid. When nucleotides are added or removed, the grouping shifts and the code for all amino acids downstream is altered, resulting in a frameshift variant. Typically, the produced protein is ineffective. Frameshift variants include instances of duplication, deletion, and insertion.

viii. Recurring expansion: Some DNA regions contain nucleotide sequences that are repeated multiple times in succession. A tetranucleotide repeat, for instance, consists of four nucleotide sequences, while a trinucleotide repeat consists of three nucleotide sequences. A repeat expansion is a mutation that increases the number of DNA sequence repetitions. This type of variation may result in an improperly functioning protein.

What Impact Could Genetic Variations Have on Development and Health?

Each cell requires thousands of proteins to perform specific tasks at specific times and locations to function properly. Gene variants, also known as mutations, can occasionally impair the function of one or more proteins. By altering the genetic instructions for producing the protein, a variant can render it dysfunctional or prevent its production altogether. When a variant alters an essential protein in the body, it can hinder normal development or lead to disease. A genetic disorder is a disease resulting from mutations in one or more genes. Occasionally, gene variations can be so severe that an embryo cannot develop into a healthy child. These mutations occur in developmentally essential genes, frequently interfering with the early stages of embryo development. These variants are incompatible with life as a result of their extremely detrimental effects. It is essential to keep in mind that genetic disorders are caused by variants that alter or eliminate the function of a gene, and not by variations in the genes themselves, which do not cause disease. For instance, "the cystic fibrosis gene" typically refers to a specific variant of the CFTR gene that causes the disorder. The CFTR gene is present in all individuals, including those without cystic fibrosis. (Dunnen, J. T. 2011).

4.3 GENE EXPRESSION DATA

Gene expression Data is generated when information encoded in a gene is translated into protein or RNA structures that are already present and functional in the cell.

Biological Interpretation of Gene Expression Data

Numerous methods for displaying and analyzing gene expression data apply to microarray and RNA-seq experiments. Here are a few of the most popular methods.

Clustering and Heatmaps

Using a heatmap to display gene expression data is common practice. The heatmap can also be combined with clustering techniques, which pair up genes and/or samples according to how similar their gene expression is. This can help locate frequently regulated genes or biological markers associated with a particular disease (e.g, a disease or an environmental condition). Each row represents a gene, and each column represents a sample when displaying data in heat maps using a grid. The color and intensity of the boxes represent variations in gene expression, as opposed to absolute values. (Smyth, G. K.2010).

Gene Set Enrichment Analysis and Pathway Analysis

Gene set enrichment analysis, based on the functional annotation of differentially expressed genes, is a common technique for interpreting gene expression data. This is useful for determining whether differentially expressed genes are linked to a particular biological process or molecular function.

Gene Ontology, which contains standardized annotation of gene products, is frequently used for this purpose. It operates by comparing the frequency of various gene list annotations, such as differentially expressed genes, to that of a reference list (usually all genes on the microarray or in the genome). KEGG, Ingenuity, Reactome, and WikiPathways biological pathways can be enriched using comparable methods.

Common gene set enrichment and pathway analysis instruments include:

- Ingenuity (license required)
- GSEA (free)
- Reactome (free)
- DAVID (free online tool)

Factors That Affect Gene Expression

Numerous variables can affect gene expression. These factors include:

- Sex-limited inheritance: Sex-limited traits are those that are exclusive to one sex. In contrast to sex-limited inheritance, X-linked inheritance refers to traits on the X chromosome. When sex hormones and other physiological differences between males and females alter the expressivity and penetrance of a gene, the phenomenon is referred to as sex-limited inheritance, or more accurately, sex-influenced inheritance. Male-pattern baldness also referred to as premature baldness, is an autosomal dominant trait that manifests in females infrequently and typically only after menopause. (Smyth, G. K. 2010).
- Genomic imprinting: Due to genomic imprinting, the expression of genetic material varies depending on whether it was inherited from the mother or the father. The majority of autosomes contain both parental alleles. In fewer than 1 percent of instances, only the paternal or maternal allele can express a particular allele. Typically, for instance, only the paternal allele contributes to the expression of the insulin-like growth factor 2 gene.

Typically, natural effects during gamete development determine genomic imprinting. Different levels of expression of specific maternal or paternal alleles may result from DNA alterations such as methylation. A disorder may appear to skip a generation if genomic imprinting prevents the expression of the causative allele. Incorrect imprinting can result in clinical conditions such as abnormal allele activation or silencing (eg, Prader-Willi syndrome, Angelman syndrome).

Codominance

The existence of both dominant alleles has been established. Consequently, heterozygotes have a phenotype distinct from that of either homozygote. A person who, for example, has one allele coding for blood type A and one allele coding for blood type B has both blood types (blood type AB).

Chromosomal Inactivation

All but one of the X chromosomes in females with two or more X chromosomes are inactive, meaning that the majority of their alleles are not expressed. Early in foetal development, each cell in the body chooses at random which chromosome to inactivate; sometimes the X from the mother is inactivated, and sometimes the X from the father is. When one parent is responsible for the majority of X inactivation, this is known as skewed X inactivation. Once a cell is inactivated, its offspring will all have the same X inactivation. On the inactive X chromosome, however, some alleles do express. Numerous of these alleles are located on chromosomal regions that correspond to Y chromosomes (and are thus called pseudoautosomal regions because both males and females receive 2 copies of these regions). (Smyth, G. K.2010).

4.4. SINGLE-CELL DATA

Single-cell data refers to the data obtained through sequencing of individual cells to obtain genomic, multi-omics, or transcriptomic information at single-cell level.

What Is the Procedure for Sequencing a Single Cell?

Various technologies are available for single-cell sequencing.

To perform single-cell RNA sequencing, the five steps below must be carried out:

- Make a suspension of a single cell.

  To separate the individual cells in the subsequent step, you must extract a suspension of single cells from your sample.

- Divide a single cell

  We must separate the cells because each will be barcoded individually in the subsequent step. Frequently, microfluidics or FACS sorting are utilized to isolate cells.

- Barcodes and Amplification

  During data analysis, a barcode can be used to identify the cells once they have been separated. The RNA is then amplified to ensure that sufficient quantities are available for library preparation.

- Construction of NGS libraries and sequencing

  Pool the amplified RNA into a sequencing library and barcode the samples with sample-specific barcodes.

- Data analysis

  Map the raw sequencing data to the reference transcriptome for data analysis. After that, utilize specialized data analysis pipelines to analyze the data.

Even the smallest populations of cells exhibit heterogeneity. If one can analyze individual cells, they can comprehend significant changes "cell by cell" as opposed to at the population level. The ability to access data at both the single-cell and multi-cell levels enables the precise collection of vital information (Satija, R. 2019).

Why Is Single-Cell Analysis Essential?

Cells must be studied at both the multi- and single-cell levels for scientists to obtain a complete and comprehensive picture. Cell-to-cell variation occurs naturally in both healthy and diseased tissues or multicellular organisms, posing significant difficulties for drug discovery and development, diagnostics, and prognosis.

The average response of the entire population is provided by the statistical analysis of whole cellular populations, which does not accurately represent any particular cell, including rare variants. Consequently, the average of a population may obscure the response of a single cell. When attempting to create accurate disease models or comprehend patient responses to specific therapies, this level of heterogeneity presents a significant obstacle. Fundamentally, the ability to investigate and characterize rare cells is provided by the analysis of individual single cells from a heterogeneous population, which also helps to reduce biological noise.

Which Common Problems Come Up When Conducting Single-Cell Analysis?

The initial isolation and culture of a single cell is one of the most difficult challenges in single-cell analysis. Cell viability is necessary for subsequent cell growth and analysis. Since cells are typically not self-sufficient, it is challenging to culture them on their own. Interactions between cells and the environment surrounding a cell have a significant effect on it. Changed and isolated single cells are no longer in their natural environment and may react erratically to the synthetic environment. In addition, the isolation procedure may unintentionally cause cell stress, which may alter behavior, viability, and profile of the cell.

The high processing power required to analyze each cell in a population in a high-throughput manner, which requires hundreds of thousands to millions of single cells, is another disadvantage of single-cell analysis.

To understand the complexities of a cell population, analysis from all angles is necessary. Multiplexing single-cell assays, however, can be challenging because numerous analysis techniques kill the cells, resulting in unreliable results.

In diverse populations, it can be difficult to distinguish biological noise from other sources of noise. Single-cell analysis can aid in the resolution of this issue in conventional assays.

As platforms and methods for single-cell analysis advance, the amount of data generated increases dramatically. It can be challenging to analyze the data produced by a single cell. Single-cell sequencing, for instance, generates massive amounts of data that require bioinformatics experts to analyze and interpret. Connecting the major phenotypic or molecular response can be challenging for the majority of data. (Satija, R. 2019).

What Measures Can Scientists Take to Address These Issues?

New technologies for delicately isolating cells are being developed to aid in the preservation of cell viability. The Cyto-Mine® Single Cell Analysis System (Sphere Fluidics) and other microfluidic platforms employing picodroplet technology to shield individual cells from shear stress are examples. The ability to perform multiple tests or continuous monitoring on a single cell can shed light on its dynamic changes. In single-cell analysis, artificial intelligence may also be able to identify data trends, which could aid in early disease detection diagnostics.

Examples of Single-Cell Technology Applications

Numerous industries benefit from comprehending the nuances of a single cell or have needs for populations derived from a single clone, adding to the extensive list of applications.

Biologic production requires single cells, which is a fundamental requirement in biopharmaceutical research and development. The International Council for Harmonization of Technical Requirements for Pharmaceuticals for Human Use (ICH) has mandated that biologics come from a single clonal source to ensure consistency and quality of production, reduce population heterogeneity, and minimize genomic instability. Similarly, induced pluripotent stem cells should be derived from a single progenitor so that the population has the same genetic background.

Identification of rare cells from large heterogeneous populations is one of the most important applications of single-cell technology. As a result, rare, valuable B cells for antibody discovery and high-expressing single cells for cell line development can be identified and isolated. This expedites entry into the supply chain for biologics. In addition, single-cell analysis in diagnostics can detect circulating tumor cells that are present in extremely small numbers and are concealed among millions of leukocytes and red blood cells in peripheral blood.

Utilizing single-cell technology has significantly increased our knowledge of the gut microbiome. The ability to identify specific functions of gut bacteria through single-cell sequencing of microbial cells may shed light on how diverse microbial strains influence disease. The same holds for environmental applications such as microbial screening in the ocean and soil remediation, as well as the search for particular traits in rare soil bacteria. If the "right" microbes are discovered for a variety of applications, this source may prove useful.

Other applications include precise genome editing, the use of synthetic biology to generate useful clones, and the investigation of cell-cell interactions to better comprehend disease mechanisms or discover new targets. (Satija, R. 2019).

Single Cell Identification Methods Available Today- Benefits and Drawbacks

- Single-cell imagers: Typically, fluorescent or colorimetric probes are used to scan single cells or cell populations for the presence of specific proteins or cell characteristics. They are useful for identifying phenotypes despite being frequently very slow and costly.

- Single-cell sequencing: After bioinformatic analysis, single-cell sequencing yields data-rich results that provide a comprehensive understanding of gene expression heterogeneity throughout a population. Only a few hundred cells per experiment are analyzed, making the throughput quite low. When combined with microfluidics, the throughput can be increased to tens of thousands; however, this is still quite low in comparison to other methods.
- Flow cytometry: Approximately 70,000 events per second are measured by flow cytometry, a well-known technology with phenomenally high throughput. There are available assay capabilities. In contrast, cell secretion assays cannot be conducted with certainty because any secreted molecule has the potential to diffuse into the extracellular environment. Although cold capture secretion assays do not provide real-time results, they do provide information about the surface-remaining secreted proteins. Flow cytometry also has the disadvantage of requiring prior knowledge of the object by labelling the target cell or object before processing. Additionally, fragile primary cells may be lost due to the high shear forces employed during sorting.
- Microfluidic droplet technology: Microfluidic droplet technology permits miniature assays and high-throughput single-cell analysis. The droplet provides a micro-reaction chamber that traps secreted antibodies and other biomolecules, enabling ultra-sensitive and rapid assays.

Integration of droplet technology into user-friendly platforms can be challenging. Cyto-Mine® is a fully automated platform that combines single-cell screening, sorting, dispensing, imaging, and clone verification using Sphere Fluidics' patented picodroplet technology. It analyzes and isolates up to 40 million cells per day that produce a specific antibody or protein, streamlining processes and increasing throughput in cell line development and biologics discovery. (Satija, R. 2019).

4.5. PROTEOMICS DATA

Proteomic data is information obtained by systematically identifying and quantifying the entire protein complement (the proteome) of a biological system (cell, tissue, organ, or organism) at a given time. Mass spectrometry is the most prevalent technique for proteomic analysis.

During the discovery of a marker, bioinformatics analyses employ novel proteomics algorithms to manage the vast and diverse data generated. It is still challenging to manage this vast amount of data and identify connections among the various omics technologies (like metabolomics and genomics). The processing parameters, quality evaluation, and lack of data format standards make it difficult to analyze proteomics data. Significant difficulty exists in the ability to analyze massive amounts of data and produce actual biological understanding. Protein pathways are cellular processes with a particular biological impact. There are many available protein pathway tools and databases. Metabolism, signaling, and interactions are extensively covered by the Kyoto Encyclopedia of Genes and Genomes, BioCarta, Pathway Knowledge Base Reactome, and Ingenuity pathway databases. GenMAPP and PanTHER are two distinct databases for protein analysis based on evolutionary relationships that have been developed to study signal transduction pathways. Databases such as Netpath, which contain cancer-related pathways, have been created to assist researchers in locating proteins specific to a particular type of cancer. Complex protein interactions are described in databases like BioGRID, IntAct, MINT, and HRPD. The STRING database contains links to a large number of additional databases for literature mining and protein interaction. In addition, protein networks can be constructed with the STRING database using the provided list of genes and interactions.

Proteomics in Medicine

Proteomics is a cutting-edge method used in medicine, such as the discovery of drugs and biomarkers. Proteomics can identify and track biomarkers by examining proteins in bodily fluids such as urine, serum, exhaled breath, and spinal fluid. Proteomics can also aid in drug development by providing a detailed map of protein interactions linked to disease pathways. (Christoforou, A. 2014).

Biomarker Discovery

A biomarker is an observable indicator of a normal or abnormal biological state in the body. Cancer biomarkers are used in clinical settings to monitor cancer progression and response to treatment. 2D-PAGE is used in the discovery of biomarkers. It can also distinguish between the protein profiles of healthy and diseased cells, including tumor tissues and bodily fluids. Cancer biomarkers are classified into three types based on their intended applications: diagnostic, prognostic, and predictive. Predictive biomarkers can predict the outcome of therapy. Tratuzumab response in breast cancer, for example, can be predicted based on human epidermal growth factor receptor 2 activations and positivity. Furthermore, mutations in the Kirsten rat sarcoma virus gene in colorectal cancer can predict treatment resistance to epidermal growth factor receptor inhibitors (e.g., cetuximab).

Prognostic biomarkers, on the other hand, can provide doctors with a prediction of clinical outcomes. The 21-gene repetition mark, for example, predicts breast cancer relapse and complete survival in node-negative, tamoxifen-treated breast cancer. The third type of biomarker is diagnostic biomarkers, which reveal whether a patient has a specific disease condition. A stool DNA test, for example, is used as a diagnostic biomarker for colorectal cancer. These biomarkers have been found in urine, blood, serum, and tissues. Body fluid sampling for proteomics is thus less invasive and less expensive. The discovery of biomarkers has aided in the treatment of a wide range of diseases, including renal disease, cancer, diabetes, cardiovascular disease, and acquired immune deficiency syndrome. However, the highly complex protein mixtures and the wide range of protein dynamics present challenges in fluid sampling for proteomics. Every type of sample has a different application depending on the disease conditions. In kidney disease, urine proteins, which represent changes in kidney functions, are evaluated using a urine sample. Blood is also used to identify biomarkers for various human diseases. Some of the challenges associated with using plasma in biomarker discovery include protein dynamicity, patient variability, and the low abundance of biomarkers in plasma. These challenges in biomarker discovery have yet to be Overcome. Because of their clinical importance, cancer-related diseases receive the majority of attention in biomarker discovery studies. There are numerous biomarkers associated with tumors, for example, that can be used to monitor patients. (Christoforou, A. 2014).

Pharmaceutical Research

Drug discovery is a multi-stage, complex process involving chemical, functional, and clinical proteomics methods. The application of proteomics in drug discovery has expanded to include patient treatment and care. 2-DE cannot be used in drug discovery because it cannot separate the membrane proteins that characterize approximately 50% of significant drug targets. Furthermore, 2-DE cannot detect low-abundance proteins. Understanding the role of proteins in a mixture and their interactions is critical for drug discovery proteomics. These techniques should also be capable of detecting low-abundance proteins and their activity. As a result, phage proteins have been identified and separated using various technologies such as MS and protein chip. Other methods, such as activity-based assays and two-hybrid assays, can also be used to achieve the same result. Using 2D-PAGE-MALDI-TOF/TOF, *Lavandula angustifolia* was used as a medication to treat Alzheimer's disease in rats.

Oncology

Oncoproteomics is the application of proteomics to the treatment of cancer. Oncoproteomics can be used to find anticancer medications and tailor cancer treatment. Microarrays and laser capture microdissection (LCM) of tumor tissue can be used to classify proteins in cancer. Oncoproteomics is used in a wide range of tissues, including the colon, breast, rectum, prostate, and brain. Proteomics can also be used to detect cancer and discover novel treatments. To find cancer biomarkers, a variety of proteomics methods such as aptamer-based molecular probes, cancer immunomics, tissue microarrays, nano-proteomics (to isolate autoantibody signatures), and antibody microarrays can be used.

LCM and MS imaging are two tumor proteomics strategies that can be used (MSI). LCM can separate the target proteins from the 'internal regions of a tumor before MS analysis. This method, which employs the "proteinChip SELDI" system, can also aid in identifying proteins that correlate with tumor progression in both the early and late stages of the disease. However, because of the technical challenges and low throughput of tumor tissues, they are used in fewer studies than serum.

The second strategy employs MSI. This direct tissue technique allows for the use of a fresh piece of the tumor and a small amount of MALDI matrix mixed. This method can be used to create three-dimensional maps of proteins and small molecules. This method was used to map 42 lung tumors alongside eight normal lung tissues. Furthermore, MSI is capable of organizing 85% of nodal connections, classifying lung cancer histology, and predicting diagnosis.

Leukemia

Proteomics enabled the discovery of numerous leukemia biomarkers capable of distinguishing between different types of leukemia. These biomarkers include catalase, annexin 1, alpha-enolase, annexin A10, tropomyosin, tropomyosin 3, peroxiredoxin 2, and RhoGDI2. These biomarkers aid in the diagnosis and progression of the disease. Furthermore, by utilizing leukemia proteomics profiles, the proteomics approach can aid in the development of new therapeutic pathways. The fact that key proteins controlling critical cellular components are present in low abundance and may be difficult to detect is a significant limitation of this approach.

The majority of early AML proteomics studies used bone marrow and peripheral blood cell samples. However, one study did compare AML at diagnosis, remission, and relapse. The proteome expression at diagnosis and relapse was found to be comparable at high protein concentrations. AML (subtypes M1 and M2) was the focus of a separate study that compared patients to healthy people. Twenty five proteins were found in bone marrow and peripheral blood samples. The M2 subtype is the only one that contains 6-phosphogluconate dehydrogenase, Annexin III, and L-plastin, according to the study. Drug resistance during relapse was found to be related to annexin I and actin gamma 1 levels.

Proteomics Controversies

Proteomics is fraught with difficulties. The main issue is that protein expression varies significantly depending on the environment and cell type. Furthermore, unlike genomics, which employs the polymerase chain reaction, proteomics lacks a comparable method. The fact that protein activities are post-transnationally highly regulated complicates proteomics. Finally, sample types and sample preparation methods are two other proteomics challenges that can significantly affect the quality of MS data. The sample manipulation method and bio-specimen type, for example, had an effect on the protein and phosphoprotein levels in breast cancer tumor samples.

4.6: METABOLOMICS DATA

Metabolomics data is defined as information that reveals the small-molecule metabolite profiles of specific cellular processes' distinctive chemical fingerprints as a result of a systematic examination of all metabolite-related chemical processes. (Lu, L. J. (2015)

What Is Metabolomics?

Metabolomics is a rapidly evolving field that combines advanced analytical techniques for identifying and quantifying cellular metabolites with statistical and multivariant data extraction and interpretation methods. Over the last 20 years, significant progress has been made in the sequencing of a wide range of organisms. Large sums of money were also invested in developing analytical methods for examining various cell products, such as proteins, metabolites, and gene expression products (transcripts). All of these "omics" techniques, including genomics, transcriptomics, proteomics, and metabolomics, are regarded as critical tools for understanding the biology of an organism and how it responds to environmental cues or genetic perturbations.

Given that metabolites "act as a spoken language, broadcasting signals from the genetic architecture and the environment", metabolomics is thought to provide a direct and immediate functional readout of physiological state of an organism. Metabolite analyses on various organisms, tissues, or fluids have been performed using a variety of analytical technologies. Mass spectrometry combined with various chromatographic separation techniques, such as liquid or gas chromatography or NMR, are the primary tools for analyzing multiple metabolites at once.

Despite the highly developed and sensitive technology of metabolomics, there are some technical challenges. Because of the enormous diversity of chemical structures and the vast differences in abundance, no single technology can be used to examine the entire metabolome. A variety of complementary approaches must be developed to extract, detect, quantify, and identify as many metabolites as possible.

Finding information in the massive amounts of data produced by high-throughput analyzers, as well as understanding it in a biological context, are additional challenges in metabolomics. Aside from being an exciting and challenging learning experience for biochemists, the use of sophisticated statistical and multivariant data analysis tools, such as cluster analysis, pathway mapping, comparative overlays, and heatmaps, has also demonstrated that current thinking needs to change to deal with large data sets and distinguish between noise and genuine sample-related information. Furthermore, the metabolomics community is still debating how to deal with data that do not make biological sense based on literature and common knowledge.

We have only begun to speculate on where metabolomics and other 'omics technologies will lead us: will they help us find more answers to our questions, or will they raise new ones that will require more answers? (Lu, L. J. 2015).

Potential Applications of Metabolomics

Target analysis, metabolite profiling, metabolomics, and metabolic fingerprinting are the four conceptual approaches to metabolomics. Target analysis has been utilized for many years to identify and quantify a small number of known metabolites (targets) using the most effective analytical technique for the compounds of interest. In contrast, metabolite profiling seeks to investigate a broader range of chemically known and unknown compounds. Using GC-MS, this strategy has been applied to numerous biological systems, including plants, microbes, urine, and plasma samples. Metabolomics employs complementary analytical techniques, such as LC-MS/MS, GC-MS, and/or NMR, to identify and quantify as many metabolites as possible, both known and unknown compounds. Metabolic fingerprinting (or footprinting for external and/or secreted metabolites) is the fourth conceptual strategy. Creating the mass profile or metabolic "signature" of a sample and comparing it to a large sample population in search of sample differences. When signals that distinguish between samples are detected, the metabolites are identified, and the biological significance of the compound can be clarified, drastically reducing the amount of time required for analysis.

Due to the close relationship between metabolites and phenotypes, metabolomics has a wide range of applications, including phenotyping genetically modified plants, testing for significant equivalence, determining how genes function, and monitoring organisms' responses to biotic and abiotic stress. Consequently, metabolomics can be viewed as bridging the gap between genotype and phenotype, providing a more comprehensive understanding of how cells function and identifying novel or striking changes in specific metabolites. To discover new biotechnological theories and targets, it is possible to mine and analyze metabolomic data sets and their metadata (Lu, L. J. 2015).

Evolution and Metabolomics

The majority of evolutionary research to date has involved the construction of phylogenetic trees of species using sequences of genomes, genes, mRNA, and/or proteins. Nevertheless, there is a weak correlation between gene expression and protein expression and an even weaker correlation between gene expression and metabolite expression. To protect themselves from potentially hazardous environments or predators, the majority of organisms rely heavily on metabolites, particularly secondary metabolites. Although primary metabolites involved in central metabolism can be used to determine nutritional and growth status, secondary metabolite profiles may more accurately reflect species differentiation and their complex responses to the environment and other organisms. Secondary metabolites are found in a wide variety of organisms, and while some of them are shared, the vast majority are highly species-specific. Consequently, secondary metabolites are considered possible phylogenetic and taxonomic markers. Smedsgaard and Nielsen (2006) have outlined the most efficient and intriguing applications of metabolomics tools for distinguishing between fungal species. Utilizing direct infusion electrospray mass spectrometry, rapid chemical classification of filamentous fungi was performed (DiMS). Various subspecies' crude fungal extracts were directly injected into a mass spectrometer, and the resulting mass profiles were analyzed using chemometric tools. Using conventional phenotypic identification as opposed to mass profile classification, more than 80% of the analyzed species could be identified.

4.7 EPIGENETICS DATA

Epigenetic data is the result of research into how changes in your environment and behavior can affect how your genes function. While epigenetic changes are reversible and do not alter your DNA sequence, they can affect how your body interprets a DNA sequence.

How Epigenetics Work

Different modifications to the epigenome affect gene expression. Modifications include:

- DNA Methylation: DNA is methylated when a chemical group is added to it. This group is commonly added to specific DNA regions to prevent proteins from attaching and "reading" genes. Demethylation is a technique used to eliminate this chemical group. Typically, methylation "turns off" genes, whereas demethylation "turns on" them.
- Histone modification: DNA is encircled by histone proteins. When histones are densely packed, the gene is "turned off" because the proteins that "read" the gene have difficulty gaining access to the DNA. Uncompacted histones permit proteins that 'read' genes to access more exposed or unwrapped DNA, thereby activating the gene. Histones can be chemically altered to become more or less densely packed, thereby activating or deactivating genes.

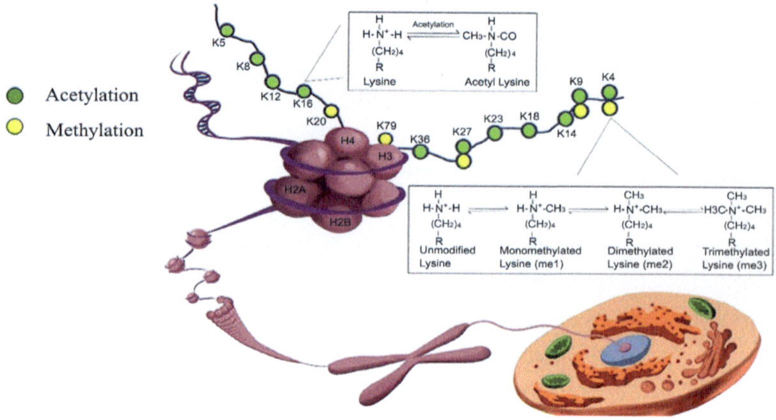

Figure 4.3: Schematic presentation of a nucleosome. A nucleosome functions as the fundamental packing unit of chromatin, with a stretch of double-stranded DNA wrapped around a histone octamer of two H2A–H2B dimers and a (H3–H4) 2 tetramer. Different possible histone modifications (mainly acetylation and methylation) at core histones and the processes of the modifications are shown.

Source: He, H., Hu, Z., Xiao, H. et al. The tale of histone modifications and its role in multiple sclerosis. Hum Genomics 12, 31 (2018). https://doi.org/10.1186/s40246-018-0163-5

- Non-coding RNA: NA, both coding and non-coding, is produced using DNA instructions. Coding RNA is required for protein synthesis. Non-coding RNA regulates gene expression by interacting with specific proteins and coding RNA to degrade the coding RNA, thereby preventing it from being used to produce proteins. To "turn on" or "turn off" genes, non-coding RNA may recruit proteins to modify histones.

Epigenetic modifications can have several effects on health:

1. Illnesses: Pathogens can weaken the immune system by altering the epigenetics, of an individual. Consequently, the germ can survive. Example: *Mycobacterium tuberculosis*

Mycobacterium tuberculosis causes tuberculosis. As a result of infection with these pathogens, a subset of immune cells may undergo histone modifications that "switch off" the IL-12B gene. When the IL-12B gene is silenced, the immune system is weakened, and *Mycobacterium tuberculosis* has a greater chance of surviving.

2. Carcinoma: Some mutations increase the likelihood of developing cancer. Certain epigenetic modifications increase the likelihood of developing cancer. For instance, if you have a mutation that prevents the BRCA1 gene from functioning normally, you are more likely to develop breast and other cancers. Similarly, increased DNA methylation increases the risk of developing breast and other cancers by reducing the expression of the BRCA1 gene (4). Although some genes in cancer cells have greater DNA methylation than in healthy cells, the DNA methylation levels of cancer cells as a whole are lower. Even cancers of the same type can have distinct patterns of DNA methylation. Epigenetics can be used to identify the type of cancer a patient has or to detect previously difficult-to-detect cancers. Because epigenetics alone cannot diagnose cancer, additional screening tests would be required to confirm a cancer diagnosis. For example, colorectal cancer.

In colorectal cancers, abnormal DNA methylation near these genes affects gene expression. Commercial colorectal cancer screening tests using stool samples, may look for abnormal levels of DNA methylation at one or more of these DNA regions. It is essential to understand that a colonoscopy is required to complete the screening process if the test result is positive or abnormal.

3. Dietary Needs During Pregnancy: The environment and actions of the pregnant woman, such as whether she consumes a healthy diet, can alter the epigenetic make-up of the fetus. Some of these changes in the child may last for decades and may increase the risk of contracting certain diseases. A good example is the Dutch winter famine (1944-1945).

During the famine, those who were carried by their mothers were more likely to develop heart disease, schizophrenia, and type 2 diabetes. Sixty years later, researchers examined the methylation levels of individuals whose mothers were pregnant during the famine. In comparison to their siblings who had not been exposed to famine before birth, these individuals had increased methylation at some genes and decreased methylation at others. These methylation variations may help to explain why these individuals had an increased risk of developing certain diseases later in life.

CHAPTER 5

TOOLS FOR DNA ANALYSIS

CONTENTS

5.1 INTRODUCTION

The interpretation of genetic sequences is made possible by DNA analysis, which is conducted for various objectives. It may be used to distinguish between species and individuals within the same species. It is expected that the DNA sequences of different animals will vary. During this time, animals may still exchange significant amounts of DNA. Humans and bananas share almost 50% of their DNA!

The bands in black-and-white photographs that resemble barcodes are one of the most well-known uses of DNA analysis. This combination of bands produces a "genetic fingerprint" that may be used to compare samples. Each of these bands corresponds to a distinct DNA fragment. This process can be used to validate or refute the biological relationship of a person to their purported father or to match the DNA of a suspect to a crime scene DNA sample. (Speed, 2012).

Before DNA testing became a viable option, criminal investigators routinely collected fingerprints at crime sites. It was believed that if thieves donned gloves or cleaned their hands, they would easily avoid detection. DNA may nevertheless be found virtually everywhere. Thieves have a far more difficult time avoiding leaving biological residues such as saliva, hair, sweat, skin, earwax, and mucus behind.

Midway through the 1980s, when DNA analysis became accessible, these biological samples were utilized in criminal investigations. Alec Jeffreys, an English scientist, created DNA profiling, sometimes known as genetic fingerprinting, to match suspects to crime scene evidence. Since then, technology has improved significantly, decreasing the cost of DNA analysis, improving its accessibility, and enabling its usage in a vast array of official and consumer applications.

DNA analysis begins with the extraction and purification of DNA from biological material. Typically, the approach utilized is dictated by the size of the sample and the predicted amount of DNA. DNA may be retrieved using a variety of methods and sources.

When doing a home DNA test, a saliva sample or cheek swab is nearly always required; the cheek swab technique is quick and painless. Numerous treatments, including prenatal DNA testing, may require a small quantity of blood. Depending on the type of sample you select, you will get a collection kit in the mail after purchasing the test. This collection kit will include all of the necessary instruments and instructions for returning the sample to the lab (Speed, T. P. 2012).

Massive volumes of biological data are created due to the use and development of cutting-edge molecular biology technology; this data must be reviewed, processed, and evaluated. In this newly developing transdisciplinary field, information from several disciplines, including biology, computer science, genetics, physics, and mathematics, are combined. Numerous informatics tools have facilitated the study of gene expression, genome exploration and annotation, and the prediction and identification of specific regions, such as promoters and splicing sites. Some of these applications can also function as web servers. On the other hand, many image analysis and processing techniques have vastly improved and have several uses, notably in the field of biology. DNA fingerprinting, a genetic typing technique that enables DNA pattern comparison and the evaluation of genomic relatedness across samples, is an extremely valuable tool in this field. Multiple firms may employ this strategy (medical diagnosis, forensic science, parentage testing, the food industry, and agriculture, to name a few). Determining the genetic similarity between several clinical isolates of bacteria is one of the most difficult elements of infectious disease molecular epidemiology. Ribotyping, rep-PCR, simple sequence repeats, RAPD, amplified fragment length polymorphism, restriction fragment length polymorphism, and pulsed-field gel electrophoresis are examples of applicable molecular techniques. Regarding the latter, it enables the separation of large DNA molecules in an agarose gel matrix through a regular shift in the direction of the electric field. It is particularly useful for tracing major clones or discovering closely related bacterial strains during epidemic follow-up due to its enhanced selection power. This is the most efficient approach for molecular epidemiology research.

Comparing patterns from a distance or visually interpreting banding patterns can be challenging and subjective at times. Several technological options are available to expedite this process and reduce human suggestibility. A researcher can, for instance, examine lanes with multiple bands and display the data in various dendrogram forms.

Despite the significance of DNA fingerprinting and the availability of numerous methodologies, there is no comprehensive comparison of the criteria addressed by each technique.

5.2. ANNOTATION

Annotation is a subset of genome analysis, which refers to everything that may be done computationally with genome sequences. Before submitting a genome sequence to GenBank and describing it in a published work, annotation is a phase of genome study that is routinely conducted. We use the word "typically" since the type of study published in the scientific literature for various genomes and the annotations made accessible through GenBank vary significantly. Publications on the human genome sequence contain a large amount of information that goes beyond typical genome annotation. The "unit" of genome annotation is a description of a single gene and its protein (or RNA) product, with the major emphasis of each record being the function of the gene product. The record may include a brief description of the evidence for this assigned function, such as the percentage of identity with a functionally defined homolog or the domain boundaries determined through a domain database search.

Annotation of the genome must involve some form of automation. Nobody will manually enter each of the thousands of protein sequences in a genome into the BLAST window, press the button, and then wait for the results to arrive on the screen. Each genome study utilizes a unique set of approaches to achieve this. Software that can do such repetitive activities in batch mode and organize data from several apps is important for annotation to be beneficial. Genome annotation, however, remains essentially "manual" (or, more precisely, "expert"), as human judgments on how to assign gene functions are made afterward (supposedly, experts). There have been several attempts to go beyond simple data processing and give a computer program full decision-making capacity.

Genomes, the fundamental unit of genetic material in molecular biology, are made of DNA. Even though the genome contains both coding and non-coding regions, the coding regions are of special importance to humans since they directly affect vital life processes. DNA includes all of the biological information necessary for the development and maintenance of an organism. Gene annotation is the process of assigning importance to a nucleotide sequence. It is a significantly lengthier method involving many stages and a vast array of actions (Ence, D. 2012).

Gene annotation refers to the process of adding layers of analysis and interpretation to the raw DNA sequence obtained through genome-sequencing research to extract physiologically relevant information and contextualize the gathered data. Using software that incorporates bioinformatics, such difficult jobs may be completed. The Institute for Genomic Research created the first gene annotation software system in 1995, which was used to sequence and study the genes of the bacteria *Haemophilus influenza*.

The process of gene annotation determines gene locations and coding areas. Annotation of genes allows us to comprehend what these genes accomplish in the body by identifying structural characteristics and linking them to the actions of various proteins. Currently, the procedure is automated, and records may be retrieved through the National Center for Biomedical Ontology database (Ence, D. 2012).

Annotation of genes can be performed manually or electronically utilizing a variety of tools created by various organizations. The disadvantages of the manual procedure are that it is time-consuming and has a poor turnover rate. However, it still has predictive value and hence serves a secondary purpose. The technique for gene annotation consists of three basic steps:

Non-coding sections of the genome have been discovered (exons). It is inefficient to devote time and effort to regions that produce little to no biological information; consequently, it is essential to restrict the scope of the study and focus just on the most crucial sections.

Gene prediction provides an overview of the amino acid segments of genes and their roles. This procedure, also known as gene discovery, identifies genomic DNA areas that contain genes. It may be accomplished by ab initio or empirical approaches.

Establishing a connection and correlation between the materials detected and the submitted biological data allows biological processes to be linked to data.

Homology-based tools, for instance, BLAST, have significantly simplified gene annotation, making it considerably easier to perform than manual techniques requiring human ability.

Genomic research has been subdivided into structural genomics, functional genomics, and comparative genomics to better comprehend this crucial subject. Gene annotation consists of two phases: structural and functional gene annotation.

Molecular weight differences, overall shape, and physical appearance are used to identify genes in the early phases of gene annotation. Changes in coding sections, gene architecture, ORFs, their positions, and regulatory motifs are a few examples of the information generated by this method that influences gene identification and differentiation. Specificity and accuracy may be used to measure the accuracy of a procedure. Specificity refers to the proportion of correctly anticipated signals among those that are expected, whereas sensitivity refers to the proportion of correctly predicted signals among all possible suitable intensities.The process of linking genetic components is displayed at the stage of structural annotation with considerable biological activity. DNA annotation frequently considers biochemical activities, physiological roles, regulating mechanisms, and interconnections on top of expressions.

Biological investigations and *in silico* analyses that simulate internal conditions may be utilized in the aforementioned procedures. Proteogenomics is a revolutionary approach for enhancing genomic annotation that uses mass spectrometry data on expressed proteins (Ence, D. 2012).

We intend to obtain CDs, mRNA, pseudogenes, promoter and poly-A signals, mRNA, and other essential information throughout the annotation procedure. These components are tiny, making their identification difficult. The technique has been aided by software and technologies created by scientists. Commonly used tools include ORF detectors, promoter detectors, and start/stop codon identifiers. Due to the dynamic nature of gene sequencing, automation has increased precision, but there are still substantial disparities between it and manually done procedures.

Expected outcomes of a successful gene annotation technique include publication, storage in a database, and dissemination for research purposes. (Ence, D. 2012).

There are still many possible uses to be identified for the brand-new and incredibly fascinating notion of gene annotation. Numerous groups have thankfully invested in gene annotation, and fresh findings are produced every day. Ensemble, GENCODE, and GeneRIF are currently active gene annotation programs. It is essential to note that new material on this topic is released every day; therefore, it is essential to remain current.

Complete gene annotation is a milestone development since it describes organisms. Annotation of DNA reveals the majority of the information contained in genomes.

Accuracy of Genome Annotation, Sources of Errors, and Some Thoughts on Possible Improvements

It is quite difficult to evaluate the accuracy of genomic annotation. Numerous studies have demonstrated that using more advanced methods for sequence comparison, such as gapped BLAST and later PSI-BLAST, which is sometimes used in conjunction with threading, as well as various types of motif analysis and careful manual integration of the results generated by all of these approaches, significantly improves the detection of homologs.

Nonetheless, genome annotation is primarily about functional prediction rather than homolog identification, making it impossible to create a truth standard. Functional annotation, or more specifically, functional prediction, focuses on proteins whose functions are, by definition, unknown, and the pace of experimental confirmation of predictions is sluggish. We believe the following method might be used to construct a test that objectively evaluates the correctness of genome annotation. It is conceivable to anticipate particular active centers and other functionally significant places for as many proteins as possible by analyzing the protein set included in a freshly sequenced genome. When a new genome becomes available, especially one that is phylogenetically distant, the orthologs of the proteins from the original genome are identified, and the conservation of the projected functional locations is evaluated. This is a tough test that would determine the lower limit of accuracy because, first, functional site prediction may be somewhat inaccurate; however, the function of the protein would still be properly predicted, and second, certain active sites in the new genome may be disrupted. A failure to preserve would constitute an error. On this basis, the accuracy of the prediction might be evaluated, and a "tournament" comparable to the CASP competition for protein structure prediction could theoretically be created (Ence, D. 2012)

Reviews of the consistency of annotations of the same genome done by various parties, as well as several "sanity checks" and expert opinions, have essentially constituted the entirety of genome annotation accuracy evaluations to date. The smallest of the sequenced bacterial genomes, *Mycoplasma genitalium*, was the subject of an interesting comparison of three different annotations, which was published by Steven Brenner. Without attempting to identify whether annotation was "better," he analyzed each contradictory annotation meticulously, removing small semantic inconsistencies and marking seeming irreconcilable ones as mistakes (in at least one of the annotations). He determined that at least 8% of the 340 genes identified by at least two of the three studies included errors. In a similar experiment employing the COG database, we observed that 194 of the 786 COGs that did not include paralogs (as of the end of 1999) had inconsistent annotations in GenBank. the use of the same criterion as Brenner anticipates a more gloomy annotation error rate of at least 25%. Even the smallest of these estimations is a significant barrier to genome annotation, raising the possibility of a catastrophic mistake event. Before providing solutions, we quickly discuss the most prevalent causes of mistakes. In the section on the accuracy of sequence database information, the most common issues encountered during human and automated genome annotation were previously covered. Even some automation of the annotation process raises the chance of all of these mistakes.

5.3. SIMILARITY SEARCHING

Utilizing sequence similarity searches to identify homologous sequences is one of the earliest and most instructive phases of evaluating newly discovered sequences. Due to the vast size of modern protein sequence databases, greater than 80 percent of metagenomics sequencing samples frequently exhibit significant similarities with proteins in sequence databases. Numerous commonly used similarity search tools, such as BLAST, PSI-BLAST, SSEARCH, FASTA, and the HMMER3 algorithms, provide accurate statistical estimates, ensuring that protein sequences with structural similarity share that similarity. Due to the possibility that sequences with a high degree of similarity are homologous, or share a common ancestor, similarity searching is both efficient and reliable. (Bajorath, J. 2011).

Inferring Homology from Similarity

Homology, or shared evolutionary origin, is essential to the study of DNA and protein sequences. On the other hand, the relationship between homology and similarity is widely misinterpreted. Homology is generated when two sequences or structures resemble one another more than chance would predict. The most plausible explanation for their striking similarities is that the two sequences evolved from a common ancestor as opposed to independently. Due to shared ancestry, a high degree of resemblance suggests a common ancestry (alternative theories call for comparable structures to evolve independently).

Even though many homologous protein alignments are unquestionably homologous based on statistically significant structural similarity or high sequence similarity to an intermediate sequence, homologous sequences do not always share strong sequence similarity. In light of this, we may be persuaded that two sequences are homologous if a similarity search returns a statistically significant match; nevertheless, if no statistically significant match is detected in a database, we cannot be positive that there are no homologs. False positives (non-homologs with substantial scores; Type I mistakes) are reduced when applying sequence similarity search strategies like BLAST, FASTA, and HMMER; however, they are not eliminated (homologs with non-significant scores; type II errors). As will be demonstrated in further detail below, locating distant homologs is often assisted by utilizing a smaller database (between 100,000 and 500,000 items) compared to the largest sequencing sets (more than 10,000,000 protein entries). Likewise, a protein domain annotated in databases like InterPro and Pfam will exist forever. However, these databases might not be able to annotate a domain if it exists but is extremely far from any known homologs (Bajorath, J. 2011).

Because excessive similarity causes homology, we must employ a statistical model to determine whether or not an alignment similarity score would be expected by chance. There are millions of useless sequences in the currently accessible big protein databases. Since the similarity scores of unrelated sequences are identical to those of random sequence alignments, it is simple to calculate the distribution of scores expected by chance. The extreme value distribution describes the expected distribution of similarity scores by chance when local sequence alignments are generated by BLAST, Smith-Waterman, or FASTA, and the scores are normalized to account for the scaling of the scoring matrix and the length of the sequences being compared (scores for alignments between two random or unrelated sequences). To convert the bit score provided by the vast majority of similarity algorithms into a probability, use the formula {p (bx) 1exp (mn22)1}, where m and n are the lengths of the compared sequences. This alleviates worries about normalization. Since the probability p (b) quantifies the likelihood of the score in a single pairwise alignment, BLAST, FASTA, and SSEARCH do not supply it. As a result, BLAST and other algorithms provide the expected frequency with which the score would occur by chance following hundreds of thousands or millions of searches. This is the expected value, sometimes referred to as value or E ()-value. After hundreds of thousands to tens of millions of comparisons, the best results are produced by the current search algorithms. E () yields E (b) p (b) D, where D is the number of sequences in the database.

Because the predicted value varies with database size, an alignment score derived from a database containing 10,000,000 items will be 100 times less significant than one derived from a database containing 100,000 entries. This does not imply that a sequence exists only in one occurrence (the smaller search). The sequences are homologous if the alignment was significant in the smaller (and shorter) search; however, the bigger search may overlook this homology since 100 times more sequences may randomly yield high (but inconsequential) alignment scores. Nonetheless, the absence of a significant similarity (in a single search) does not always imply the absence of homology. Homologous sequences have a high degree of resemblance to one another. When alignments are insignificant, homology can be established by comparing to an intermediate sequence, employing profile- or HMM-based methods, or both. Due to the possibility that sequences with a high degree of similarity are homologous or have a common ancestor, searching by similarity is efficient and trustworthy. Despite its simplicity, it may be challenging to comprehend how to compare biological facts. The majority of DNA, RNA, and protein sequence databases are large, complicated, and multi-dimensional. Theoretically, simple techniques such as dynamic programming and heuristic solutions fail to align numerous sequences. The best features of both systems may be combined in a breakthrough method based on advancements in computer science that would deliver exceptional performance without losing accuracy (Bajorath, J. 2011).

DNA sequence comparison rather than protein sequence comparison is the most typical cause of missing homologs (or translated DNA sequences). DNA: DNA searches are considerably less sensitive compared to protein (and translated-DNA) searches. Protein: protein or translated DNA: protein alignments have an evolutionary look-back duration five to ten times longer than DNA: DNA alignments. In contrast, protein alignments frequently show homology between sequences that last had a common ancestor more than 2.5 billion years ago (e.g., humans to bacteria). Moreover, whereas protein: protein alignments with expectation values of 0.001 may be used to reliably infer homology, DNA: DNA alignments with expectation values of 106 are more likely to occur by chance, and 1010 is a more widely accepted threshold for homology based on DNA: DNA searches. Instead of DNA: DNA alignments, the most effective strategy for boosting search sensitivity using DNA sequences is to employ translated-DNA: protein alignments, such as those created by BLASTX and FASTX.

For valid homology conclusions, dependable statistical estimations are necessary. The statistical evaluations offered by BLAST, FASTA, SSEARCH, and other well-known similarity search techniques are very trustworthy. In rare circumstances that may look scientifically intriguing, however, statistical estimation fails, and unrelated sequences are ascribed statistical significance not owing to homology but rather due to statistical faults. When a scientifically unexpected alignment appears to be statistically significant, researchers should investigate a variety of methods for determining significance. Statistical estimates can be confirmed in one of two ways: by doing more searches with scrambled copies of the original sequences, or by attempting to identify the most comparable alignments to unrelated sequences and determining that such alignments are insignificant. Since it is difficult to identify with certainty that two sequences are unrelated, particularly when unexpected homology inferences are made, strategy (1) may appear troublesome. On the other hand, alignments with high scores that result by chance might be highly changeable as they do not reflect evolutionary links. The structure and domain classifications of unrelated sequence alignments will vary considerably. Since sequence alignments with proteins containing unrelated domains must be unrelated, the domain structures (and potentially structural classes) of high-scoring alignments can be utilized to discover the highest-scoring unrelated sequences. Correct statistical estimations indicate that unrelated sequences (sequences from separate domains) will have E ()-values of 1; if unrelated sequences have E ()-values of 0.001-0.01, the scientifically new link is questionable.

The second technique, which employs randomized sequences of identical length and composition to infer relevance, is more straightforward; however, it relies on the premise that randomized sequences have characteristics with authentic protein sequences. This is true for the great majority of sequences, but the assumption may be less accurate in exceptional situations that produce "new" outcomes. The most effective shuffling algorithms preserve the local amino acid composition by inverting one of the sequences or by shuffling the sequences in local windows of 10 or 20 residues. SSEARCH and the other applications in the FASTA software suite generate statistical estimates based on shuffles that preserve local composition.

The statistically significant similarity in a BLAST, FASTA, SSEARCH, or HMMER search can be used to infer homology (shared ancestry and similar structure), but this does not indicate that every protein component is identical. BLAST, SSEARCH, FASTA, and HMMER are used to construct local alignments of sequences; they reveal the regions of two sequences that are most similar. For proteins with a single domain, the conclusion of the alignment may match the termini of the protein.

However, for proteins with multiple domains found in different sequence contexts, the alignment should only include the homologous domain, since this homology contributes to the sequence similarity measured by the score (Bajorath, J. 2011). The sites at which local alignments within a protein terminate might vary depending on the scoring matrix used to generate the score. Scoring matrices such as BLOSUM50 and BLOSUM62, which are used by SSEARCH, FASTA, and BLASTP, and BLOSUM62, which is used by BLASTP, are intended to identify extremely distant similarities and have very low penalties for mismatched residues. A homologous area that shares at least 50% of its components with neighboring non-homologous sections may thus grow. This is a common source of mistakes in iterative methods such as PSI-BLAST, although it may be mitigated by limiting extension in subsequent rounds (Bajorath, J. 2011).

Searching for Similarity in Biological Sequences Is Challenging

Finding patterns in biological data is a crucial step in several data analysis methods used in the life sciences, including omics analysis. Finding meaning entails recognizing similarities and differences. Whether they are creating evolutionary trees, identifying conserved domains in proteins of interest, or investigating structure-function connections, from DNA to RNA to amino acids, they all rely on a few methodologies to uncover similarity and dissimilarity in biological sequences.

Assigning regions of high similarity against high variation and matching letters on a grid are the fundamental problems in locating and aligning sequences. However, nature has significantly contributed to the difficulty of this undertaking.

Due to the three billion base pair size of the human genome, sequence similarity searches are rarely restricted to a straightforward one-to-one query. This is the initial issue posed by the sheer volume of data. In big genome sequence datasets, genomic sequence alignment yields n-on-n searches. The basic act of matching letters on a grid of this size is labor-intensive; consequently, shortcuts may hide vital informative sequence data.

In addition to being enormous, biological sequencing data is notoriously difficult to manipulate when doing alignment searches. In biology, data is continually changing. Errors occur each time DNA replication begins. Errors are possible when a gene is transcribed, or a transcript is translated.

The propensity for mistake at the core of life is believed to molecularly fuel the ability of living things to adapt to their environment. This sophisticated technique for repetitive adaption enhances the complexity of biological data. It is challenging to distinguish "natural noise" from significant changes in biological data resulting from random mutations and other oddities (SNVs, CNVs, inversions, etc.).

The convergence of all these traits in biological datasets presents conceptual and analytical difficulties. Even the most elementary instance of recognizing a DNA pattern in a biological database is not mathematically well-posed. This suggests that there may be more than one possible answer.

Sequence Alignment: Dynamic Programming Is Slow but Reliable

There are several approaches to solving the sequence similarity search problem. Given a collection of query strings, each seeks the most similar or identical units, often bases or amino acids (of any kind).

Dynamic programming is the initial method for sequence alignment. In contrast, dynamic programming is computationally inefficient and should only be utilized for alignments of two, three, or four sequences. In other words, scaling is not possible with these options. In the 1970s and 1980s, the Needleman-Wunsch and Smith-Waterman approaches for sequence alignment were developed (Homer, N. 2010).

Typically, the first phase of a dynamic programming methodology is to generate alignment spaces for each pair of input sequences. This produces a collection of one-on-one alignments, which are subsequently integrated into an n-level alignment grid, where n is the number of query sequences. Dynamic programming is time-intensive, yet it consistently yields the best outcomes.

In contrast to heuristics, dynamic programming techniques do not "cut corners," making them the best option for aligning a small number of sequences. Dynamic programming is also simple to implement with open-source Python toolkits such as Bio Python, which includes the Bio.pairwise2 module for fundamental pairwise sequence alignment and additional modules for more complex alignments.

Sequence Alignment: Heuristics Are Fast but Cut Corners

Heuristics are pragmatic approaches to data problems that do not produce ideal results. In other words, a heuristic method may not provide an alignment that accurately represents the degree of sequence similarity. Even though this looks to be a stern warning — after all, who wants a less-than-desirable outcome? — This is not the case. Heuristic algorithms are substantially less computationally costly than dynamic programming techniques due to their pragmatic nature.

Complex multiple alignment problems can only be solved via heuristics, as traditional dynamic programming approaches would need days or weeks of computation time.

FASTA, which was created in 1985 and proved popular for sequence alignment almost immediately, was followed by BLAST in the 1990s.

Utilization of word techniques or k-tuples is the primary achievement of these heuristics. These algorithms construct "words" by matching short sequences from the sequence query with other sequences in a database. By using these words to generate an initial alignment, sequences may be offset, resulting in a relative position alignment that significantly accelerates the remaining sequence alignment procedure.

Notably, the FASTA approach is distinct from the FASTA file format, which has become the industry standard in bioinformatics for DNA, RNA, and protein sequences, as well as the default input format for FASTA alignment software (Homer, N. 2010). Numerous sequence alignment algorithms use progressive techniques, which begin by matching the two most similar sequences and then add progressively fewer similar sequences to the grid until all sequences are included. The initial selection of the "most similar sequences" using this technique is significantly weighted, which is a drawback. The final alignment will be inaccurate, if the initial estimate of which sequences are most closely related is inaccurate. Clustal and T-Coffee are two prevalent progressive heuristics methods.

A New Gold Standard: The Need for Optimization and Indexing

Both dynamic programming and heuristics-based solutions have been studied in the past; however, neither is flawless. The first may overlook vital information, while the second lacks the processing efficiency of a truly scaled instrument. As database complexity rises and data analysis quickly becomes a bottleneck in many pipelines, a tool that combines the advantages of dynamic programming and heuristic approaches while avoiding their limits is urgently required. Utilizing strategies from contemporary computer science, such as optimization and indexing, is one answer to this issue. Although hidden Markov models excel in matching distantly related sequences, they are often inferior to more established techniques such as dynamic programming and heuristic approaches. The indexing procedure, on the other hand, uses Google-like techniques to identify brief meaningful patterns in biological sequencing data, which are then abstracted and indexed for rapid retrieval at all molecular levels.

By not providing a pre-selected search window while employing this approach, bias is avoided. A simple case study describing the search for resilient domains in the variable region of immunoglobulins utilizing HYFTs TMpatterns, which enable ultra-fast, ultra-precise sequence alignment, is described below (Homer, N. 2010).

Case Study: Finding Robust Domains in the Variable Region of Immunoglobulins

Immunoglobulins, often known as antibodies, are adaptable, therapeutically useful proteins with a vast array of uses in illness detection and treatment. Antibody monoclonal treatment is increasingly used to treat complex diseases such as cancer.

The identification of sequence similarity in the immunoglobulin variable region is essential for the development of these medications. Although this problem may be solved using heuristics or traditional dynamic programming, the former performs poorly, and the latter may result in the loss of binding sites owing to a restricted search window. Using HYFTS-pattern-based indexing algorithms, the whole sequence is quickly searched.

The immunoglobulin protein sequences in the PDB have been reduced to HYFTS patterns, which provide quick abstractions of searchable sequences. All sequence outputs are then aligned based on their HYFTS patterns. The method creates 900 non-identical sequences aligned in the constant region (red) of the immunoglobulin and with higher variety in its variable section (blue). A brief search finds multiple conserved domains in regions widely believed to be very variable, indicating that the variable region is not entirely random.

This fast, parameter-free search exemplifies the potential of index-based sequencing alignment methodologies for bioinformatics, and it may become the industry standard shortly. It took less than a second and required no preprocessing or parameter adjustments. Even though there are several solutions to the sequence alignment problem, the most used dynamic programming, and heuristic methodologies still have design flaws. Due to advances in computer science that emphasize indexing and optimization, the efficiency and accuracy of sequence alignment algorithms are projected to increase significantly.

Due to the significance of research into methods for assessing similarity across biological sequences during the past decade, several computational and statistical approaches have been developed for comparing biological sequences. The computational biology research community faces a substantial challenge in this regard. There are two main bioinformatics methods for detecting the similarity or dissimilarity of sequences: alignment-based and alignment-free procedures. Large biological datasets present a computational obstacle for discovering optimal solutions utilizing sequence alignment-based methods. Research into alignment-free sequence analysis is increasing to circumvent the multiple severe restrictions of alignment-based sequence analysis.

5.4. MOLECULAR EVOLUTION

Molecular Phylogeny of Genes

Since the 1980s, systems for identifying DNA nucleotide sequences have undergone substantial development and automation. Numerous genomes, including those of viruses and humans, have been sequenced due to a large number of genes and a variety of species. Utilizing DNA sequences has greatly assisted the study of gene duplications. Hemoglobin-coding genes in humans and other animals are a good example.

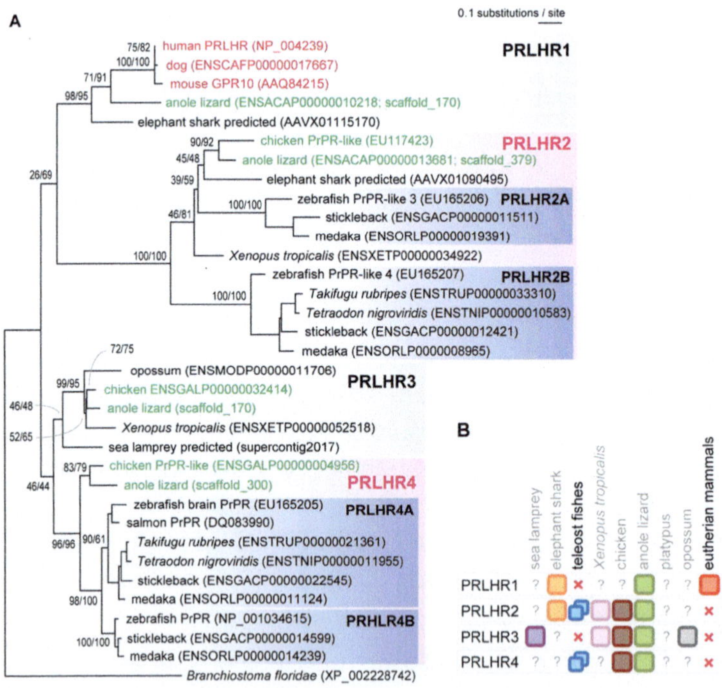

Figure 5.1: Molecular phylogeny of PRLHR genes. (A) The molecular phylogenetic tree was inferred with the ML method (a 5 0.85; 228 sites). Genes of sauropsids (birds and reptiles) are shown in green, and those of eutherian mammals are shown in red. Support values shown at the nodes are bootstrap probabilities in the ML and neighbor-joining (NJ) trees in that order. The chicken PRLHR2 gene (PrPR-like gene; EU117423) is found only as a transcript in Ensembl, but seems to contain an intact open reading frame. Vertebrate subtypes

containing gene losses are shown with pink shading. (B) A schematic illustration of the absence and the presence of multiple subtypes of PRLHR genes. For mammals and teleosts, in which we confirmed gene absence with multiple sequenced genomes, gene absence is indicated with ''Â.''

Source: Genome-Wide Detection of Gene Extinction in Early Mammalian Evolution - Scientific Figure on ResearchGate. Available from: https://www.researchgate.net/figure/Molecular-phylogeny-of-PRLHR-genes-A-The-molecular-phylogenetic-tree-was-inferred_fig4_51807175 [accessed 25 Nov 2022]

Due to similarities in the amino acid sequences of hemoglobin chains and the myoglobin protein, it is now possible to reconstruct the evolutionary history of the gene duplications that gave rise to the relevant genes. A detailed examination of the nucleotide sequences of the genes that produce these proteins indicates that the situation is far more complex and intriguing than the protein sequences suggest.

DNA sequence analysis indicates that human hemoglobin genes contain more genes than previously believed. Hemoglobin molecules are tetramers composed of four subunits consisting of two polypeptides of one kind and two polypeptides of a different type.

Fetal hemoglobin F, adult hemoglobin A, and adult hemoglobin A2 are known to contain one of the two kinds of polypeptides. Hemoglobin A comprises around 98% of adult human hemoglobin, but hemoglobin A2 comprises barely 2%. What additional sort of polypeptide is present in hemoglobin in adults, fetuses, and embryos? On chromosome 11 are genes that code for the first set of polypeptides, while on chromosome 16 are genes that code for the second group. (Sironi, M. 2017).

There are still further difficulties to overcome. Two genes (named G and A) and two extra genes are present (known as 1 and 2). A pseudogene, two pseudogenes (1 and 2), and a pseudogene are also present (numbered 1 and 2). Due to the presence of termination codons and other mutations, these pseudogenes are incapable of producing functional hemoglobin.

Since the polypeptide genes and pseudogenes in the gene families have identical nucleotide sequences, they are homologous, indicating that they originated from a single gene through gene duplication and subsequent evolution. Moreover, the nucleotide sequences used to differentiate between genes are virtually similar. The evolution of the genes responsible for producing myoglobin and hemoglobin.

Multiplicity and Rate Heterogeneity

Only 104 amino acids are represented by 312 nucleotides in cytochrome C. Nonetheless, this little protein has a plethora of evolutionary knowledge, allowing scientists to reconstruct the history of 20 extraordinarily varied species spanning over a billion years, as seen in the picture. Cytochrome c, on the other hand, is a slow-changing protein. It is feasible to investigate genetic differences across distantly related creatures since many of the amino acids in their cytochrome c are derived from vastly dissimilar species. Comparing cytochrome c molecules cannot demonstrate evolutionary relationships between closely related species. Even though humans and chimpanzees split around 6 million years ago, their amino acid sequences remain comparable. Humans and rhesus monkeys diverged from their common ancestor between 35 and 40 million years ago by a single amino acid change.

Proteins that increase at a quicker rate than cytochrome c can be investigated to determine the evolutionary links between closely related species. Fibrinopeptides, which are required for blood clotting, can be used to reconstruct the phylogeny of recently developed animals, such as closely related mammals. Hemoglobin, for instance, can be utilized to recreate the evolution of species over a very long period. Other proteins evolve more gradually.

There are hundreds of genes and proteins in each organism, each of which represents the same evolutionary events but evolves at a different rate. By analyzing new genes, researchers may recreate the evolutionary tree of any collection of species with better precision. Various gene sets may be studied to achieve varying degrees of clarity in the tree while depending on slower-changing genes for distant evolutionary events because genes evolve at different rates. Examining redundant codon substitutions (nucleotide substitutions that do not alter the encoded amino acids), introns (non-coding DNA segments interspersed with segments that code for amino acids), or other non-coding segments of the genes can be used to reconstruct the evolutionary relationships between closely related species, even if the genes encode proteins that evolve slowly (such as the sequences that precede and follow the encoding portions of the genes) (Sironi, M. 2017).

The Molecular Clock of Evolution

A crucial aspect of molecular evolution is the ease with which changes between homologous molecules may be detected and quantified, for example, by the number of nucleotides or amino acids that have undergone mutations. Consequently, DNA or proteins can be employed to estimate rates of evolutionary change more precisely than phenotypic form and function characteristics. Studies of the rates of molecular evolution inspired the notion of macromolecules functioning as evolutionary clocks. The distance between any two species from a common ancestor revealed in the 1960s seemed comparable to the number of amino acid differences between homologous proteins of those two species. Proteins and DNA sequences would serve as a molecular clock of evolution if the rate of evolution of a protein or gene was almost constant along the evolutionary branches that lead to diverse species. The sequences may, therefore, be used to recreate the date and order of each evolutionary branching event.

Below is the phylogeny of twenty unique species. If the rate of nucleotide substitution in the gene-producing cytochrome c remained constant across time, we could measure the length of time that has passed along each branch of the phylogeny by counting the number of substitutions. For the clock to accurately depict the geologic time that has passed in at least one lineage, it must be calibrated using an external source, such as the fossil record.

In contrast to a watch or other precise timepiece, the molecular evolutionary clock is designed to be a stochastic clock, similar to radioactive decay. In a stochastic clock, the probability of a given amount of change is constant, but the actual amount of change might vary (for instance, a specific number of radium-226 atoms is expected to decay to half in 1,620 years). Over extraordinarily large time intervals, the precision of a stochastic clock is rather good. The molecular evolutionary clock is extremely promising since each gene and protein has its own time. Even if each gene and protein evaluates the same evolutionary events differently, each clock "ticks" at a pace proportional to the average rate of evolution of the relevant gene or protein.

According to evolutionary experts, the observed diversity in DNA and protein evolution is greater than what a stochastic clock would predict, supporting the unexpected nature of the clock. Nevertheless, differences in evolutionary rates between lineages are minimal. It is theoretically possible to precisely plan evolutionary processes since the clock is stochastically constant; nevertheless, twice as many genes or proteins must be analyzed. When several species are examined, and long-term evolutionary processes are observed, the average rates recorded for specific proteins give a very accurate clock (on the order of 50 million years or longer). Evolutionists have demonstrated that molecular time estimations are often older than those derived from other methodologies and sometimes older than the dates themselves. This is because of the irregular distributional characteristics of molecular estimates. Depending on chance, the number of molecular differences between two species may fluctuate significantly. Overestimation errors cannot reach zero, and neither can underestimation errors. Consequently, a graph representing the usual age range at which two species diverged based on many genes is skewed, with a huge cluster of younger ages at one end and a long "tail" of older ages trailing toward the other. Consequently, the average of the estimated durations will never match the actual date. When the rate of molecular evolution is slower, the sequences employed are shorter, and the period is longer, the overestimation bias is more prominent.

The Neutrality Theory of Molecular Evolution

In the late 1960s, it was believed that genetic drift, not natural selection, drove the majority of molecular-level evolutionary changes that happened selected "neutrally." Mutations alter the amino acids and nucleotides of a population.

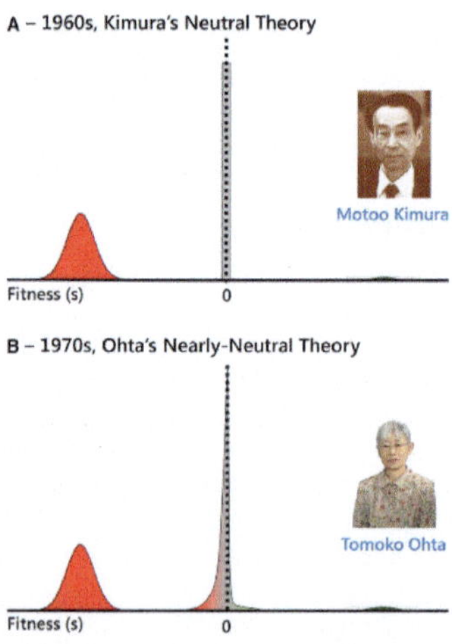

Figure 5.2: DFE according to the (nearly) neutral theory of molecular evolution. (A) In the 1960s, according to the neutral theory of Kimura. (B) In the 1970s, after the extension of the neutral theory by Ohta. Different selection coefficients of mutations are colored in a gradient from maroon (strongly deleterious), red (slightly deleterious), gray (neutral), light green (slightly advantageous), and dark green (advantageous).

Source: Molecular Population Genetics - Scientific Figure on ResearchGate. Available from: https://www.researchgate.net/figure/DFE-accord-

ing-to-the-nearly-neutral-theory-of-molecular-evolution-A-In-the-1960s_fig4_314281390 [accessed 25 Nov, 2022]

Only if distinct alleles (differing DNA sequences) were equally fit or capable of executing their assigned purpose would their frequency vary between generations. For a particular gene or protein, allelic substitution rates will be stochastically constant or occur with a constant probability. This graph depicts the rate of mutation for neutral alleles. The majority of possible mutations at each gene locus, according to the neutrality theory, are harmful to human health. Evolutionary theory suggests that natural selection should eradicate these mutations. According to the neutrality theory, morphological, behavioral, and ecological characteristics evolved due to natural selection. Each gene locus has several beneficial mutations that are almost identical, and hence, resistant to natural selection. Random genetic drift determines which mutations gain prevalence over time in one or more species. Changes in the frequency of neutral alleles are induced by random drift rather than natural selection due to their modest fitness differences. This concept is quantified by Equation 4Nes 1, which measures the fitness discrepancy between alleles. Ne represents the effective population size, whereas s represents the selection coefficient.

Assume that k represents the neutral allele replacement rate throughout evolution, represented as a rate per interval of time. As temporal units, years or generations may be utilized. In a population of N diploid individuals generated by random mating, $k = 2Nux$, where u is the rate of neutral mutation per gamete per unit of time and x is the chance that a neutral mutant will be fixed. Since the chance of 2Nu mutations per unit of time is constant, it is simple to construct this equation. All 2N genes in a population of N diploid individuals have the same likelihood of being fixed, $x = 1/(2N)$ if they are all fixed, assuming neutrality (2N). If this value of x is inserted into the preceding equation ($k = 2Nux$), the solution is $k = u$. According to this theory, population size and other environmental factors do not affect the rate of neutral allele replacement and mutation.

If the neutrality hypothesis of molecular evolution is accurate, there should be a molecular evolutionary clock, as neutral mutations should occur consistently over evolutionary time and across numerous lineages. Therefore, the diversity of amino acids and nucleotides between species only reflects the length of time they have been separated.

Divergent opinions exist among evolutionists on the feasibility of the neutrality theory. Research into the molecular clock has discovered that molecular evolution rates vary far more than predicted by the neutrality hypothesis. Other investigations have uncovered a substantial difference between the genetic diversity seen in populations of a single species and that predicted by the concept. According to proponents of the theory, these differences can be addressed by slightly modifying the primary premise, such as supposing that alleles are predominantly neutral but have tiny variations in selection value. The "null hypothesis" or starting assumption of neutrality theory serves as the basis for computing molecular evolution.

CHAPTER 6

TOOLS FOR RNA ANALYSIS

CONTENTS

6.1 INTRODUCTION

It is critical to quantify gene expression and identify transcripts that differ in their levels of expression in two different conditions in a cell, tissue, or organism to understand the molecular physiology of the cell. RNA-seq analysis using next-generation sequencing (NGS) data is now the de facto method for analyzing gene expression across the entire transcriptome. This analysis is frequently required to develop mechanistic hypotheses about molecular events in cells and tissues. Cellular responses to physiological stimuli are one example, as are the effects of experimental perturbations on specific genes and pathways and gene regulation dysfunction in disease. Total RNA is isolated from target tissues or cells for RNA-seq, which then involves creating DNA libraries from these libraries and sequencing them with a next-generation sequencing machine (Smyth, G. K. 2014).

Transcriptomics experiments have frequently measured the RNA levels expressed in tissues or cells from virtually any organism. This method has been used since the introduction of Northern blot hybridization analysis, and the advancement of microarray technology has allowed it to be scaled up. To measure gene expression at the genome-wide level, RNA sequencing (RNA-Seq) experiments have recently replaced microarrays, improving transcriptomics. As a result, microarrays or RNA-Seq technologies have generated massive amounts of data, necessitating the development of ad hoc methods to fully analyze and compare gene expression for a given organism across various conditions, tissues, and cell populations.

To quantify transcription levels and identify differentially expressed genes using RNA-Seq data from high-throughput sequencing technologies, the workflow described here can be followed:

- RNA-Seq read quality evaluation FastQC is a high-throughput sequence data quality control tool (Babraham Bioinformatics) FastQC: A High-Throughput Sequence Data Quality Control Tool (Babraham Bioinformatics)
- Filtering or trimming of reads
- Connecting filtered/trimmed reads to a reference (genome or transcriptome)
- Compiling the read count for each gene
- Differential expression analysis

Due to the size of the datasets, the user must complete steps 1 through 4, but numerous tools are available for each step that have been extensively used and cited elsewhere. The differential expression analysis, on the other hand, is most likely the critical step that allows the user to comprehend the biological data about the expression profiles of a specific organism under various conditions.

The gene expression profile contains information about genes involved in an organism's response to a specific condition. To retrieve this data, differential expression analysis must be performed, and statistical techniques are required to distinguish between expression changes caused by the tested conditions and biological "noise" or variability. Several computational tools are currently being developed, mostly written in the R programming language. These packages can be found in the Bioconductor project repository. However, the R language and packages are primarily used through a UNIX-based operating system and command-line instructions, which require some programming expertise.

As a result, to use differential expression tools, non-bioinformatics researchers must use either a graphical user interface (GUI) or web-based applications. For a GUI-based solution, a local installation of every package required for differential expression analysis is still required, which may be difficult. Web-based applications are currently emerging as a better option for performing differential expression analysis in a more user-friendly manner and without the need to install software on a local computer. (Smyth, G. K. 2014).

6.2 GENE EXPRESSION ANALYSIS

Microarrays, which allow scientists to track the expression of tens of thousands of genes simultaneously, are driving the biotechnology revolution. Regardless of the platform or analysis techniques used, the most common outcome of a microarray experiment is a list of genes discovered to be differentially expressed. Researchers must be able to translate such lists of differentially regulated genes to understand the underlying biological phenomena better. The first step in this direction can be the translation of the list of differentially expressed genes into a functional profile, which can provide insight into the cellular mechanisms relevant to the given condition. To assist with this task, a method for automating ontological analysis using Gene Ontology (GO) was proposed in 2002. (Khatri et al., 2012). Between 2003 and 2005, 13 additional tools for this type of analysis were proposed, and new tools are still being developed daily. This methodology is currently used for secondary analysis of high throughput experiments, and numerous tools have been developed for this purpose. Although these tools share a general approach, they differ significantly in many areas, which significantly impacts the results of the analysis. Most of the time, scientists using these tools must be aware of certain critical features.

Comparison of Existing Functional Profiling Tools

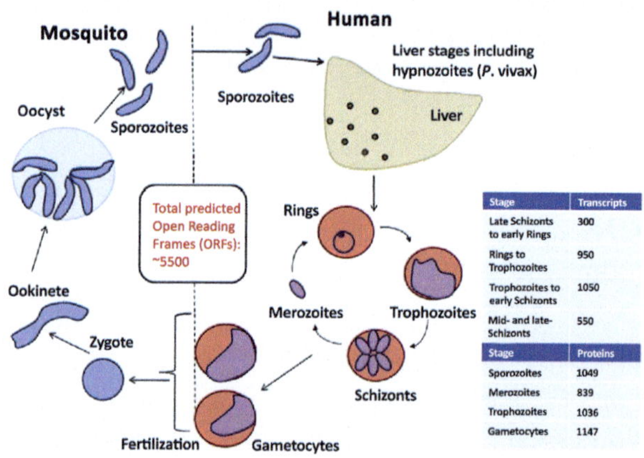

Figure 6.1: Plasmodium life cycle and expression of transcripts and proteins at different stages of the life cycle.

Source: Narayan, Kumar, Singh, Babar, Chaudhari, Patankar, 2012. Regulation of gene expression in Plasmodium falciparum.

A detailed comparison of the tools currently available for the ontological analysis of high-throughput gene expression experiments is provided below.

The Statistical Model

Statistical models such as hypergeometric, binomial, X^2 (chi-square), and Fisher's exact test can be used to conduct the ontological analysis. A hypergeometric distribution is an appropriate model for the likelihood that a specific category in the list of differentially regulated genes occurs x times by chance. Large arrays, such as the Affymetrix HGU133A, can make calculating the hypergeometric distribution more difficult. However, when there are many genes, the hypergeometric distribution tends to resemble the binomial distribution. (McCarthy, D. J 2010). Therefore, when larger arrays are used, the binomial model works perfectly. Alternative strategies include Fisher's exact test and an X^2 test for proportional equality. Most of the time, there will not be a big difference between the models. In the literature, these tests are covered in great detail (Drăghici, 2013). FatiGO does not employ a statistical model in the traditional sense. However, it does compute percentages about the GO-annotated genes or the entire set of known genes In an organism. Only one statistical test is supported by GoMiner, EASEonline, GeneMerge, FuncAssociate, GOTree Machine (GOTM), GOSurfer, Ontology Traverser, and eGOn. gOstat only offers two tests (X^2 and Fisher's exact test), while CLENCH and GOToolBox offer three (X^2, hypergeometric, and binomial for CLENCH, and hypergeometric, binomial, and Fisher's exact test for GOToolBox).

Group of Reference Genes

When identifying statistically significant GO terms, the reference list of genes against which the P-values for each GO term in the results are calculated is critical. A number of tools, including GOToolBox, gOstat, GoMiner, FatiGO, and GOTM, use the whole set of genes in a genome or the set of genes with GO annotations as the reference. Because genes that do not appear on a microarray will never be selected as differentially regulated, either of these options may be inappropriate when the input list of genes to these tools is a list of differentially expressed genes obtained from a microarray experiment. The basic idea is to assign significance to various functional categories by comparing the observed number of genes in a given functional category with the number of genes that might appear in the same category if a selection were made randomly from the same pool. If the entire genome is used as the reference, the pool considered when determining the random choice includes every gene in the genome. A gene not represented on the array used will never be found to be differentially regulated, so the pool available for selecting differentially regulated genes is limited to those represented on it. This contradicts the underlying assumptions of the statistical models used. (McCarthy, D. J 2010)

Adaptation for a Variety of Experiments

The correction for multiple experiments is an important part of evaluating a functional category. This type of correction must be made whenever a functional category is not chosen a priori and multiple such categories are considered at the same time. Nonetheless, some of the tools examined here, such as GoMiner, DAVID, GOTM, CLENCH, and eGOn, do not perform such a correction.{Re = (nf/n)/(Nf/N)}, where nf and Nf are the numbers of genes in the functional category of interest in the selected and reference sets, and n and N are the number of genes in the selected and reference sets, respectively, yields a "relative enrichment" statistic. Although this relative enrichment is somewhat redundant but less informative than the P-value, it cannot be used to account for multiple experiments; rather, it serves as another indicator of the significance of the given category. This statistic may be misleading, because the user may be tempted to interpret all enriched categories in biological terms. Any particular relative enrichment value has a non-zero chance of occurring by chance. Instead of relying on relative enrichment to determine whether a category is significant or not, the magnitude of the probability should be considered.

All the remaining tools address the issue of multiple comparisons in some way. GeneMerge and EASEonline both support the Bonferroni correction. Bonferroni and Idák are ideal in many situations, particularly when not many functional categories are involved (e.g., fewer than 50). These corrections are considered overly conservative when more categories are included, as described by Drăghici (2003). The Holm step-down family of methods allows for less conservative P-value adjustments. For this type of analysis, statistical techniques such as Bonferroni, Idák, and Holm's step-down adjustment make the well-known false assumption that the variables are independent. When dependencies are known to exist, Benjamin and Hochberg (1995) believe that false discovery rate (FDR) techniques are more appropriate. Bootstrapping is another effective strategy for calculating the null distribution by performing numerous resamplings from the same data and accounting for all existing dependencies. Extreme caution should be used when only a few categories are involved because the number of distinct resamplings may not be enough to draw a definitive conclusion. In those cases, even Bonferroni or idák may be preferable to bootstrapping. (McCarthy, D. J 2010)

The tools that provide multiple correction techniques allow the researcher to tailor the analysis to the number of categories and the strength of their known interdependencies. Bonferroni and Idák are appropriate when only a few distantly related categories are present. Holm's may be a good compromise if more unrelated categories are involved. When several functional categories are obviously related, FDR is most likely the best option. Suppose the dependencies are very strong (for example, multiple sub-processes of the same larger process). In that case, a bootstrap or Monte-Carlo simulation approach may better capture them, but only if enough categories are present to make the simulation meaningful.

Regarding this criterion, FuncAssociate is the only tool that uses a more novel Monte-Carlo simulation. FatiGO and gOstat implement Holm's and FDR corrections. Unlike GOToolBox, which provides FDR, Bonferroni, Holm, Hochberg, and Hommel corrections, Onto-Express provides FDR, idak, Holm's, and FDR corrections.

The Scope of the Analysis

When assessing the utility of a tool, it is critical to consider whether it can provide a complete picture of the phenomenon under research. When performing functional profiling using GO, the three main GO categories that should all be included in a complete analysis, along with any additional data that may be available, are Molecular function, biological process, and cellular component. The tools examined that only analyze one category at a time are eGOn, FatiGO, GeneMerge, and Ontology Traverser. The user can use other tools to analyze all three categories simultaneously. Both GeneMerge and Onto-Express have additional features. GeneMerge displays metabolic and signaling pathways from fruit flies and yeast, as well as information on yeast deletion viability. Onto-Express also displays KEGG signaling pathways and the chromosomal location of genes with differential regulation. (McCarthy, D. J 2010)

Visualization Capabilities

A directed acyclic graph is a hierarchical structure that looks like a tree (DAG). Unlike a tree, a DAG allows a node to have multiple parents. Because the DAG structure tends to clutter the display, it may not be the best option for GO navigation. A tree structure is another way to represent and visualize the DAG structure of GO, in which a node with multiple parents is represented in the tree more than once, once under each parent. Any tool that uses GO to perform functional profiling on a list of genes should be able to represent the hierarchical relationships between different functional categories.

With the help of a graphical representation of the analysis results in the hierarchical context of GO, the user can better understand the phenomenon under study. Furthermore, the functional analysis can be continued and improved by investigating a few intriguing GO hierarchy sub-graphs. Among the tools examined are DAVID, EASEonline, FuncAssociate, GOstat, GOToolBox, and OntologyTraverser, which do not display the results in the context of the GO hierarchical structure. Onto-Express, eGOn, FatiGO,

CLENCH, GoMiner, and GOTM represent the results in their GO context. GOMiner, please continue. GOTM and eGOn allow the user to collapse and expand nodes manually. Furthermore, Onto-Express supports searching and sorting within the hierarchy, expanding and collapsing nodes as needed.

Custom Level of Abstraction

In the hierarchical structure of GO, the genes are annotated at various levels of abstraction. For example, one type of "induction of apoptosis" is "induction of apoptosis by hormones," which is a subset of "apoptosis." Apoptosis has a higher level of abstraction than hormone-induced apoptosis, which has a lower level of abstraction. Every effort is made to provide the highest level of detail when annotating genes with GO terms in order to provide the lowest level of abstraction. For example, rather than simply using terms like "induction of apoptosis" or "apoptosis," a gene known to induce apoptosis in response to hormones will be annotated with the phrase "induction of apoptosis by hormones" (McCarthy, D. J 2010). The ability of a functional profiling tool to allow the user to select a specific level of abstraction is extremely valuable. This viewpoint categorizes the tools under consideration into one of three groups.

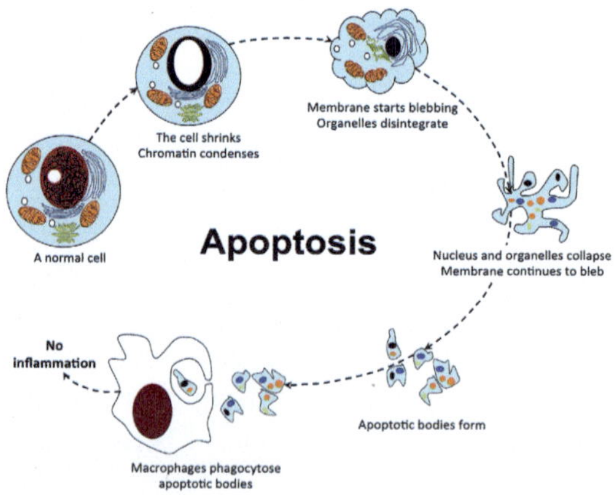

Figure 6.2: Cytology of apoptosis.

Source: Regulation of Ceramide Channel Formation and Disassembly: Insights on the Initiation of Apoptosis - Scientific Figure on ResearchGate. Available from: https://www.researchgate.net/figure/Cytology-of-apoptosis-The-different-stages-of-apoptotic-cell-death-start-by-cellular_fig3_274013152 [accessed 25 Nov 2022]

The tools in the first category can only perform analyses using the specific terms associated with each gene. This is the same as performing an analysis at the highest level of specificity or the lowest level of abstraction. This analysis consists primarily of a single search through the annotation database. Because further investigation will only yield identical results, each dataset can only be examined once. The analysis cannot be tailored in any way or tailored to answer specific biological questions.

The second type of tool allows the user to select a specific level of abstraction or depth in GO. Once this level has been selected, these tools will consider any genes associated with the corresponding category at the chosen level. To ensure that each category is propagated up through all of its parents, care should be taken to adhere to the DAG structure rather than the tree structure that may be used for visualization. The user can refine this analysis by running it at different levels of abstraction with the option to select a predetermined depth. These forces various extremely specific terms to be grouped into more general and potentially useful categories. When this is done, a number of genes that were previously classified as "positive regulation of apoptosis," for example, are now classified as "induction of apoptosis by X, Y, and Z." Because each specific category has few genes associated with it, it frequently does not appear to be significant. However, the more general category, which includes all the genes associated with the specific subcategories, is frequently found to be highly significant. The use of such tools enables a more in-depth and complex analysis that can be focused on addressing specific biological queries.

The third category includes tools that allow for custom cuts through the GO at various levels of abstraction and in various directions. For example, suppose the analysis is run at a fixed depth of 9. In that case, it can differentiate between various subtypes of apoptosis induction, such as those caused by hormones, extracellular signals, intracellular signals, and so on. However, the same analysis will be performed on thousands of additional functional categories located at the same level for a fixed depth. Suppose the results are displayed as a bar graph. In that case, the interesting categories will be obscured by all the different categories that just happened to be at the same depth in GO, even if they are not interesting to the researcher. Furthermore, other phenomena may be overlooked because the chosen level may need to be more specific for those GO categories. The most effective tool will enable the user to analyze at different depths in different parts of the GO hierarchy, as required by the biological hypothesis under investigation.

Most currently available tools analyze only at the lowest level in GO, using the same categories that genes have been annotated with, and do not allow for further refinement. Users of the reviewed tools FatiGO, EASEonline, GOToolBox, and GOstat can select a level of abstraction before submitting the input list of genes. FatiGo, CLENCH, and GOMiner assign a P-value to each node in the GO. This is equivalent to a global static analysis in which every gene under a specific node is considered to be associated with that node. At the moment, Onto-Express is the only tool that allows for completely customized analysis by allowing any GO node to be collapsed or expanded. When a node collapses, all of the genes associated with any of its descendants are reassigned to it. The P-value determined in Onto-Express for a collapsed node matches the P-value determined in the global static analysis of GoMiner and FatiGo. When a node is expanded, the genes associated with it and those associated with its descendants are identified. The P-value of an expanded node will only be based on the genes that are directly linked to it. This P-value is not available in any of the tools examined here. The current limitation of Onto-Express is that if the user wants to perform the analysis across GO at a fixed depth, they must manually expand the nodes to the desired level (McCarthy, D. J 2010).

Installation and Prerequisite Issues

Another important consideration is the effort required to install and use a tool. Web-based services provide a practical solution for experimental biologists by avoiding the issues associated with the local installation of a program. Security concerns, on the other hand, may initially prevent access to web-based tools. Before the tool can be used, the required port on the firewall must be open, for example, if it uses a specific TCP/IP port and the researcher is behind one.

Standalone tools like CLENCH, GoMiner, and GoSurfer force the user to understand the complexities of a software installation. CLENCH, for example, requires the prior installation of Perl modules for the following:

- HTTP request handling
- File and console access
- third-party gateway interface
- Database access
- Statistical analysis
- Graphical display

To view the results as a DAG and molecular structures from the Entrez structure database, for example, the user of GoMiner must install the NCBI Cn3D browser plug-in and the Adobe Scalable Vector Graphics plug-in from Adobe, respectively. However, the main GoMiner application works without the plug-ins. Web-based tools such as Onto-Express, EASEonline, DAVID, GeneMerge, Ontology Traverser, GOTM, FuncAssociate, and FatiGO require only a web browser and an Internet connection. In reality, platform compatibility issues affect even web-based tools. For example, the Microsoft Virtual Machine with the Internet Explorer browser does not fully implement the Java standard. As a result, some Java-based tools, such as Onto-Express, require the installation of the Sun Java Runtime Environment.

Two other issues are the accessibility of the tool and the requirement for an Internet connection. Web-based tools, while accessible from any computer, require an Internet connection. Although standalone tools must be installed locally on each computer from which they are to be used, they can be used without a network connection. However, once the application and the necessary data files have been downloaded, the only standalone tool in GoSurfer allows the user to analyze data without network access. The remaining standalone applications connect to local database servers (GoMiner, EASE, and DAVID) or retrieve annotation data in memory (CLENCH). These standalone tools are similar to web-based tools because the client tool requires network access to connect to the database server unless the client and the database are both on the same computer. From this standpoint, the deciding factors are specific specifications and user preferences of the application.

The most important issue in this group is version control. Because the researcher can always be sure they are using the most recent software version, web-based tools are far superior. The group that created the tool is always responsible for updating the software or database on the server. Because standalone tools must be regularly checked for new updates and releases, version control is typically the responsibility of the user. When such an update becomes available, the user is again responsible for updating the software or data, and the installation process must be repeated. Because of issues with the local environment, the updated version frequently outperforms the older version. In theory, standalone tools could solve this problem by providing automatic software updates. Because of the possibility of hundreds or thousands of different installations, this approach requires that the updating software accurately identify and deal with a wide range of local software environment issues, many of which differ slightly.

Data Sources

Most tools rely on annotation data from a single open database. The advantage is that the data is always as up-to-date as the database used. The disadvantage is that no single database can provide a comprehensive picture. The GO database is a complete and up-to-date source for primary GO annotation data because contributing databases directly commit their data there. From the standpoint of GO annotations, there is little benefit to obtaining this data from multiple sources, as other sources, such as Entrez Gene, obtain their data from the GO database. However, the secondary analysis discussed here will be more powerful if more data types are integrated coherently. A specialized annotation database that combines various types of data from various sources may be more useful than any single database (like KEGG pathways). The disadvantage of such a database is that it is difficult to create and must be updated whenever one of its source databases is updated.

This puts much pressure on the team in charge of maintaining it. Given this, it stands to reason that the vast majority of tools only use one of the annotation databases available. EASEonline, GOSurfer, eGOn, and GOTM use the GO database, whereas GeneMerge, GoMiner, and GOToolBox use Entrez Gene. Onto-Express, which uses its own Onto-Tools database, is the only current attempt to combine resources from various annotation databases. Onto-Tools currently links to and uses data from the databases GenBank, dbEST, UniGene, Entrez Gene, RefSeq, GO, and KEGG. Onto-Tools uses data from Wormbase and NetAffx without being affiliated with them.

Supported Input IDs

The probes on a microarray each identify a unique nucleotide sequence, which in turn identifies a unique gene. Annotation databases typically use genes to provide functional annotations. To create a functional profile for a list of differentially expressed genes, one must first translate the list of probe IDs into a list of genes. Similar circumstances apply when functional annotations are provided using proteins, necessitating additional gene-to-protein mapping. When using an ontological analysis tool that accepts multiple types of IDs as input, the user will not have to translate one type of ID (such as Affymetrix probe IDs) to appropriate IDs.

Onto-Translate, MatchMiner, and the Gene Name Converter are three separate Onto-Express, GoMiner, and GeneMerge tools that allow users to convert from other ID types (such as GenBank accession numbers, RefSeq

IDs, and so on) to the type(s) of ID used by the application. Although these tools can theoretically accept more types of IDs, the user must manually transfer the results from the conversion tool and submit them to the ontological analysis tool, adding another step to the analysis pipeline. For this comparison, we only considered the capabilities of the ontological analysis tool itself. (McCarthy, D. J 2010)

Only organism-specific IDs from the GO database can be entered into GoMiner, GeneMerge, and GOToolBox. Ontology Traverser, CLENCH, and FuncAssociate all accept only one type of ID. Affymetrix probe IDs, MODB gene products, and *A. thaliana* MIPS IDs are all supported by these tools. FatiGO accepts GenBank accession numbers and Affymetrix probe IDs, whereas GOToolBox accepts gene symbols and GenBank accession numbers. Onto-Express, DAVID, EASEonline, and GOTM support the most diverse types of IDs: Affymetrix probe IDs, GenBank accession numbers, UniGene cluster IDs, and Entrez Gene IDs. Furthermore, DAVID accepts GenPept, PIR, and UniProt protein IDs, as well as RefSeq IDs, whereas Onto-Express, GOTM, and other tools only accept gene symbols.

The Limitations and Drawbacks of the Current Approach

Using one or more annotation databases, each tool generates a list of function categories in which the genes from the input list are known to participate. The functional groups statistically significantly overrepresented in the list of genes with differential regulation are assumed to be meaningfully related to the condition under investigation. However, annotation databases have some significant drawbacks to converting a list of differentially expressed genes into a list of functional categories. These limitations are inherent in all available tools because they are inherent in the approach itself.

To begin with, existing annotation databases are deficient. Only a small percentage of known genes in nearly all sequenced organisms have functional annotations. Furthermore, most annotation databases are built by curators who manually review the existing literature. Even though it is unlikely, some well-known facts could be overlooked briefly. In the early 1990s, 65 functional annotations that have yet to be added to current functional annotation databases were mentioned in the literature. For example, despite being implicated in pigment biosynthesis in 1992, the gene HMOX2 is still unclassified today. The time lag required for manual curation is the primary reason recent annotations are frequently missing from databases. Second, some information may be inaccurate or untrustworthy. Among the biological process, 11 434 of the 19 490 annotations for *Homo sapiens* available in the GO are based solely on electronic annotations (i.e., without any expert human involvement). In general, these electronic annotations are fairly accurate. Because these annotations are frequently made at very high-level GO terms, their applicability is limited. Furthermore, King (2003) asserts that some of these conclusions are incorrect. Even if the error is obvious to a human expert in some cases, there currently needs to be automated techniques for examining, detecting, and correcting such incorrect assignments. Because experimentally derived annotations are more reliable than those inferred electronically, it is a limitation that none of the current tools allow for any sort of weighting based on the type of evidence.

The current method for ontological analysis is limited to searching through previously made annotations and running significance tests on the discovered categories. Even if the data support such conclusions, this method cannot reveal previously unknown functions for known genes. For example, the SLC13A2 gene (solute carrier family 13 (sodium-dependent dicarboxylate transporter), member 2 (*H. sapiens*)) encodes the human Na(+)-coupled citrate transporter, which is annotated in GO for the molecular function organic anion transporter activity. Organic anion transport, the corresponding biological process, is not annotated. This is fine for the curator, or the human expert searching GO for this specific gene. A gene encoding an organic anion transporter will be involved in organic anion transport.

On the other hand, a search that looks for every gene associated with organic anion transport will not find this gene. Similarly, suppose no other genes are involved in organic anion transport, then, any ontological analysis software attempting to determine what underlying processes are represented by a given list of genes containing this gene will either ignore it or calculate its statistical significance incorrectly by omitting it.

6.3. RNA STRUCTURE PREDICTION

RNA was once thought to be a passive carrier of genetic information, but it is now known to play a more active role in nature. Many newly discovered RNAs are catalytic, such as self-splicing introns and RNase P, which are both involved in mRNA and tRNA maturation. Furthermore, there is evidence that the presence of RNA-based organisms was required to evolve modern DNA-protein-based organisms. The number of non-coding RNAs (ncRNA) produced by humans is unknown, but research in this area suggests that it is comparable to the number of proteins produced. The surprising lack of correlation between the number of protein-coding genes and our concept of "organism complexity" has been attributed to the control of gene expression via a combination of alternative splicing and non-coding RNAs, implying that the "Central Dogma" (RNA is transcribed from DNA and translated into protein) is woefully inadequate, at least in higher eukaryotes (Weeks, K. M. 2010).

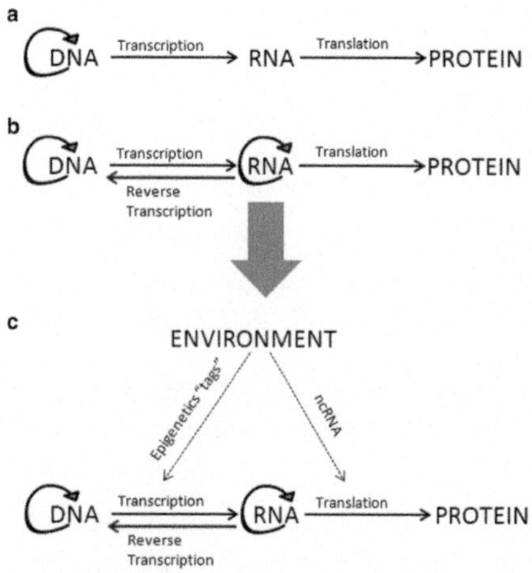

Figure 6.3: Evolution of the central dogma of molecular biology. a Most common vision in current textbooks of grade 10; b most common vision in current textbooks of grade 12; c proposed revision of the central dogma, including epigenetics. ncRNA, non-coding RNA.

Source: Exploring the Conceptual Challenges of Integrating Epigenetics in Secondary-Level Science Teaching - Scientific Figure on ResearchGate. Available from: https://www.researchgate.net/figure/Evolution-of-the-central-dogma-of-molecular-biology-a-Most-common-vision-in-current_fig1_338385911 [accessed 25 Nov 2022]

A fundamental tenet of biology is the requirement for a stable tertiary structure for biological function. In the case of RNA, the secondary structure, which is the base-pair set for an RNA molecule, supports the tertiary structure. However, scientists increasingly turn to computational techniques because experimentally determining the RNA structure is still difficult. The most widely used structure prediction algorithm is the Minimum Free Energy (MFE) method for folding a single sequence, which has been implemented by two packages: Mfold and RNAfold. In general, using comparative methods yields the highest accuracy. There are currently three methods for performing an automated comparative RNA sequence analysis, all of which are supported by comparative research. Plan A entails aligning sequences using common multiple sequence alignment (MSA) software (ClustalW, t-coffee, and PRRN) and then inferring a consensus structure using signals from structure-neutral mutations. In this situation, the mutual-information measure is frequently used. Recently, tools have been developed that combine MFE with a covariation score or probabilistic models built from large reference data sets. A step that aligns multiple sequences, on the other hand, requires a well-conserved sequence. This is only sometimes the case, as incorrect sequence alignments can eliminate any covariation signal in rapidly evolving ncRNA sequences. This has motivated Plan B, which involves using the Sankoff Algorithm to simultaneously align, fold, and infer a protosequence for a collection of homologous structural RNA sequences. The recurrences combine sequence alignment and Nussinov (maximal pairing) folding (Weeks, K. M. 2010).

To run the algorithm, extreme computational resources are required (O(n3m) in time and O(n2m) in space, where n is the length of the sequence and m is the number of sequences). Foldalign, Dynalign, and PMcomp are restricted Sankoff algorithm implementations that limit the size or shape of substructures. If no practical level of sequence conservation is discovered, the final strategy (plan C) is used. Secondary structures can be predicted separately for each sequence (or subgroup of sequences) and then directly aligned. Because of their nested branching, RNA structures are effectively modeled as trees. Similarity measurement via edit operations, a common method for string comparisons, has been extended to trees. Tree alignment and tree comparison models have been developed and implemented. Whether the initial independent folding results in at least some structures that align well, providing hints as to the underlying consensus structure, if one exists, is critical to Plan C. A growing number of researchers have recently published new RNA structure analysis and prediction algorithms. Despite this, only some algorithms are evaluated using standardized example data sets, frequently not compared to other algorithms with a similar history. Algorithm evaluation is common in protein structure prediction groups, gene prediction, and MSAs.

Consensus Structures and Structural Alignments

The prediction of base pairs that make up the *in vivo* structure using only the base sequence is known as RNA secondary structure inference. There are three general points to remember:

- In addition to the primary structure, cellular elements such as chaperones, base modifications, and the transcriptional process can affect the *in vivo* structure. There are currently no computational tools available to evaluate these effects.
- There are "riboswitches," sequences with two or more functional structures. Such cases will deceive all of the tools discussed because requesting a single consensus structure is incorrect. On the other hand, the possibility of conformational switching can be precisely identified.
- Although pseudoknots are possible in some structures, most modern tools ignore them due to their rarity and computational complexity. Pseudoknots are not considered here. However, several comparative strategies incorporating pseudoknots are currently being developed, and they unquestionably merit their comparative analysis. Remember that we frequently do not know whether the factors (1-3) apply in a given application scenario.

The comparative approach to structure inference begins with a collection of homologous RNA sequences. Attempts are made for each of them to infer the *in vivo* structure and a consensus structure that captures the shared, significant structural features. Because the consensus structure does not exist in living organisms, working with this concept necessitates some mathematical rigor.

A consensus structure lacks associated sequence information but displays base pairs shared by most structures under consideration. A concrete sequence typically contains additional base-pairs properly nested between the consensus in each structure. A structure refold (B, C) is the best thermodynamic folding for B that exhibits the base-pairs specified by C as well as others that do not contradict the former. It is made up of a consensus structure C and a sequence B that is compatible with it. The -C option of RNAfold can be used to achieve refolding (this option is used to constrain the minimum free energy prediction with prior knowledge – such as known base-pairs, unpaired regions, etc.). If there are gaps between B and S, we fill them before folding and reintroducing B and S in the same places.

Given a consistent structural alignment and the ability to count majorities at individual positions, it is simple to derive a consensus structure. Consistency implies that the 3' partner of a base-pair joins the consensus if the partner of the base-5' pair crosses the majority threshold. (Weeks, K. M. 2010).

By computing Si=refold, a structural alignment can be approximated, given a consensus structure and a sequence alignment without structural information (Bi, C). This is referred to as structural alignment reconstruction. In terms of base-pairs of C, all Si are consistent with C and one another, but they may be for something other than the base-pairs added during refolding. This is acceptable because family members only need to agree on extra-consensus features if we trust the consensus to capture the relevant common structural features.

Analyzing Data from a Database

The "truth" that we have at our disposal is not the same as that sought after by plans A, B, and C that we are about to compare. Only by way of illustration do structural databases convey agreement. They provide a reference sequence, say B1, with an experimentally proven structure S1, and an MSA of B1, S1, and additional sequences B2, Bn in the family under consideration. The sequence alignment was chosen to highlight structural similarities between the reference structure and the other family members. However, neither the specific model used to achieve similarity nor the extent to which it was optimally solved is known.

This situation may lead us to believe that the reference structure is the only reliable anchor point for evaluation. The ability of comparative analysis tools to forecast this specific structure based on family data would then be evaluated. This is a worthwhile course of action, but it ignores the impact of structural homogeneity within a sequence family and the difficulty or success of exploiting it (Weeks, K. M. 2010).

Single-Sequence Methods Have Limitations

Single-sequence prediction techniques have systematic limitations in terms of precision. The thermodynamics may be inaccurate because some parameters are extrapolated, and parameter measuring conditions *in vitro* and *in vivo* differ. The thermodynamic model estimates the actual physics of RNA folding. Furthermore, many structural RNA bases undergo chemical modifications such as sugar methylation, pseudo-uridine, dihydrouracil, and others, typically ignored by these methods. The folding kinetics are also overlooked. There is no way to separate base pairs and structural components critical for the consensus from those unique to the sequence given a single sequence. Furthermore, while some functional RNAs have bistable structures, others do not, and the optimal MFE structure has no biological significance. This provides some justification for researchers' use of comparative methods.

Comparative Method: Folding and Alignment (Plan A)

To simulate realistic RNA folding studies, we use Clustal W to re-align each test dataset and then fold them using the methods listed below. The predicted resulting structures were then compared to the consensus structures we had previously reconstructed.

- **RNAalifold**: RNAalifold uses an extension of the Zuker-Stiegler algorithm to compute a consensus structure from RNA alignments. The formula determines an averaged energy matrix

  $$\bar{E}_{ij} = \sum_{k}^{N} E_{ij}^{k}$$

  (where N denotes the number of alignment sequences) and the covariation score matrix, B ij, enhanced with penalties for inconsistent sequences. A standard trace-back procedure is used to find a consensus structure with the ideal sum-of-average-energy-and-covariation-score. The algorithm is incredibly efficient, requiring only O(Nn2 + n3) time and O(n2) memory.

  Compared to the MFE-methods, the sensitivity, selectivity, and correlation values of RNAalifold predictions were 57-91%, 57-100%, and 0.57-0.95, respectively, indicating a significant improvement in accuracy measures.

- **Pfold**: Pfold implements an RNA alignment input and generates a prior probability distribution of RNA structures using stochastic context-free grammar (SCFG). Weights are applied to posterior probabilities calculated using a maximum-likelihood phylogeny from large reference data sets.

  In general, the algorithm is accurate and efficient. As a result, the overall sensitivity, selectivity, and correlation of the Pfold predictions ranged from 0 to 100%, 0 to 100%, and 0.0 to 1.0, respectively. When empty structures (LSU rRNA (H & M) and SSU rRNA (M)) were removed, prediction accuracy ranged from 66 to 100%, 89 to 100%, and 0.77 to 1.0, respectively. The authors are working on solving the "under-flow errors" that are causing the zeros (pers. commun. Bjarne Knudsen).

- **Iterated loop matching (ILM)**: ILM, one of the few RNA folding algorithms used for comparison, can produce pseudo-knotted structures. A secondary structure is created using a combination of thermodynamic and mutual information content scores. All potential stems (including small internal loops and bulges) are generated and ranked using a combination of thermodynamic and mutual information scores. The highest-scoring stem is selected, scores are updated, stems that conflict with the selection is removed, and the next highest-scoring stem is selected. This algorithm is repeated until no stems remain. On high-similarity data, ILM performed poorly in selectivity and was less sensitive than RNAalifold or Pfold, but it improved on medium-similarity datasets. The overall sensitivity, selectivity, and correlation range of predictions by ILM were 44-100%, 37-75%, and 0.40-0.86, respectively. We re-evaluated ILM with reference structures full of pseudo-knots to ensure that the low selectivity values were not due to the reference structure lacking pseudo-knots. The new sensitivity, selectivity, and correlation values ranged from 31 to 100%, 2 to 75%, and 0.29 to 0.86, respectively; in fact, evaluating pseudo-knotted structures did not improve ILM selectivity significantly. However, remember that when a significant proportion of true base-pairs are involved in pseudo-knots, the sensitivity of the other (non-knot-inclusive) methods must decrease (Weeks, K. M. 2010).

  Because the number of secondary structures generated by incorporating pseudo-knot prediction increases significantly, they are usually not included in exhaustive folding algorithms. Furthermore, experimentally derived thermodynamic parameters like pseudo-knots are generally scarce. Because ILM is still in development, performance may improve once pseudo-knots can be more precisely modeled.

A Comparative Study of Sequence Alignment and Folding (Plan B)

Sankoff

The Sankoff algorithm employs dynamic programming to generate a list of common base pairs with the highest base pair weight sum possible. This is a hybrid of Nussinov (maximal-pairing) folding dynamic programming methods and sequence alignment. Sankoff's algorithm can produce both a consensus structure and an alignment. Full implementations of the "Sankoff algorithm" have been found to be too computationally demanding (O(n3m) in time and O(n2m) in space for sequence length n and m sequences) to be useful for the simultaneous solution of RNA folding, alignment, and protosequence problems. As a result, three constrained versions of this algorithm are now in use. Foldalign, Dynalign, and, most recently, PMcomp are examples. As a relative of the Sankoff method, we include Carnac, a recent invention that seeks to identify conserved stems in unaligned sequences.

Foldalign

According to one interpretation, Foldalign is "a combination of local alignment and the maximum number of the base-pairs algorithm." MDAs are created using pair-wise comparisons and compared using a combination of "clustal" and "consensus" heuristics. By limiting the maximum motif size (in this study, 50) and prohibiting bifurcating structures, the time complexity is reduced to O(n4N) (multi-loops). A simple match-based scoring system is used to rank putative conserved structure elements.

Foldalign is generally subject to the Tool Abuse Disclaimer because all our data sets contain multiple loops. Because Foldalign is designed specifically for the location of short regulatory motifs such as IREs, where the motifs are only related at the level of (non-bifurcating) structure rather than sequence, it is not recommended Foldalign be used to predict global, multi-looped secondary structures. This explains why our test data sets had low sensitivity, selectivity, and correlation, ranging from 5-24% to 23-36% and 0.11-0.27, respectively.

Dynalign

Dynalign implements the Sankoff algorithm pairwise, finding a common low-energy structure (including multi-loops) and aligning two structural RNAs. The computational complexity of the full Sankoff is reduced by limiting the difference between the indices I and j of aligned nucleotides (where I index positions in sequence 1 and j indexes positions in sequence 2). Furthermore, Dynalign, like MFold, reduces the conformation space by capping the size of internal loops. As a result, O represents complexity (n3M3).

The current Dynalign implementation only supports pair-wise sequence comparisons. Rather than computing all pairwise foldings, we compared all sequences to the reference structure. Due to the computational cost involved, this algorithm could only be used to predict the structures of tRNA. Dynalign performed well on the tRNA, medium sequence homology data set (sensitivity, selectivity, and correlation, averaged over all pairwise alignments with the reference sequence, were 94%, 95%, and 0.94, respectively). After removing the high-scoring point, the averaged values for sensitivity, selectivity, and correlation were 32-54%, 33-54%, and 0.32-0.54, respectively.

Carnac

The Carnac algorithm, as previously stated, is not a strict implementation of the Sankoff algorithm. A set of filters is used, with pairs of sequence sets passing through them. After scanning sequences for stems and identifying "high similarity" regions of sequences (dubbed "anchor points"), a dynamic program is used to select conserved stems using information from anchor points and covariation. (Weeks, K. M. 2010).

Alignment of Predicted Structures (Plan C)

RNA Forester

RNA forester implements the tree alignment model. In contrast to methods that only generate a similarity value with no underlying alignment, it computes pairwise alignments of two input structures. We used the global mode of RNAforester to generate global or local alignments. A branching (tree-like) structure alignment can be used to derive a set of matching base-pairs, which can then be evaluated similarly to the other approaches.

MARNA

The next step of the MARNA algorithm is to generate pairwise edge weights between nucleotides. Structure-enhanced-sequence-similarities are used to transform weights from Zhang suggested edit distances. In phase two, the alignment edges are piped into the t-coffee to produce multiple alignments. The resulting alignments are not strictly structural in the sense previously defined. Rather, these are sequence alignments influenced by structure.

CHAPTER 7

TOOLS FOR PROTEIN ANALYSIS

CONTENTS

7.1 INTRODUCTION

Proteins are a class of chemical compounds that are assembled from chains of polypeptides and amino acids. Despite their seemingly small size and complexity, they are involved in a wide variety of physiological processes that are essential to survival.

Proteins are made up of millions of smaller building blocks called subunits, which are then folded and aligned into three-dimensional structures. The process that defines this event is called protein folding. A protein is made up of twenty different amino acids, and the unique way in which these amino acids are attached is what gives the protein its distinct three-dimensional structure and, by extension, its function.

Proteins are essential for the regulation of cellular activity, the formation of tissues and organs, and the performance of their functions. They are essential to all forms of life on Earth and play a key role in the entirety of the biological sciences. Enzymes are a common type of protein that catalyze a broad variety of chemical processes and are therefore an essential component of the metabolic process. In discussions among scientists on the relationship between protein size and molecular weight, particle size analyzers are frequently used. This is because the size of the protein is an incredibly essential quantitative property (Jones, D. T. 2013).

A protein is made up of twenty different chains of amino acid residues, all strung together in a certain order. There is a minimum need for the number of amino acid residues that must be present for a biological action to be carried out, and the minimum size of a functional domain is between 40 and 50 amino acids. Multifunctional proteins can have as few as this many amino acid residues or as many as several hundred. The three-dimensional structures of many different kinds of proteins are notoriously complicated, as they are composed of hundreds of atoms arranged in a wide variety of patterns. Proteins are formed when molecules undergo a folding reaction that results in a complex three-dimensional structure. In a period that is often much shorter than a second, each protein folds into its uniquely folded form. Not only does the precise folding structure of the protein influence its function, but it also determines how the protein interacts with other molecules. A gene in the DNA of a live cell must include a precise sequence of amino acids for that sequence to be translated into a protein. Even though messenger RNA, often known as mRNA, is required for the production of proteins, it is still possible for cells to have proteins, even in the absence of mRNA. Even if there is a great deal of mRNA available, proteins can only be produced in response to the instructions that are provided by the genome. Because of this, the existence of a particular protein in a living cell at any one time has nothing to do with the mRNA that is associated with producing that protein. The production of proteins can be a challenging process. The RNA molecule is responsible for the creation of the bridge in ribosomes, which serves both as a structural support and an engine in the process of protein synthesis. Ribosomes are essential pieces of cellular machinery that are required for the production of proteins (Jones, D. T. 2013).

When researching the structures of proteins, four organizational levels need to be taken into consideration: The fundamental building block of proteins is an extensive and orderly chain of amino acids. The arrangement of amino acids in the molecule that makes up each protein is unique. "The side chain conformations of a protein are not considered part of its secondary structure, which may be thought of as the spatial arrangement of the structural components of the protein. The entire tertiary structure of the protein may be seen as having a three-dimensional form. Subunit structures of quaternary proteins consist of two or more chains of polypeptides and are found in proteins that have quaternary structures.

The amino acid residues that are the backbone of a protein are connected by peptide bonds, which can be covalent. The three-dimensional structure of a protein is held together by a variety of different types of connections and interactions, the most important of which are ionic bonds, hydrogen bonds, covalent bonds, and hydrophobic interactions. The structural components of proteins consist of domains and polypeptides, respectively (motifs). A particular area of a protein that is thought to fold and function independently from the rest of the protein is referred to as a "domain," and the word "domain" is used to designate this region. Proteins are made up of motifs, which are tiny sections that are conserved between species. Peptide bonds are formed whenever there is a condensation of two amino acids that each include an alpha-amino group. Peptide bonds are the essential structural building blocks of proteins, and proteins' primary structure is formed from these peptide bonds. When attempting to establish the identity of a protein, it is very necessary to locate the amino acid that serves as the protein's signature. To get insight into the main structure of a protein, one may make use of the resource known as PROWL. On this page, you will find information about amino acids, including their characteristics, the possible bond geometries, the probability that a particular amino acid will be an inner residue rather than an outer residue, and the amino acid substitutions that are most likely to preserve the structure and function of the protein.

Additionally, this page offers connections to additional sites that explore the application of secondary structure to the prediction of protein structure and function. Several examples of secondary structural components include the alpha helix, the beta-sheet, and the random coil. There is a variety of folding techniques, patterns, loops, and twists that may be applied. In the following part, we will discuss various software packages that have the potential to be utilized in the process of structure prediction.

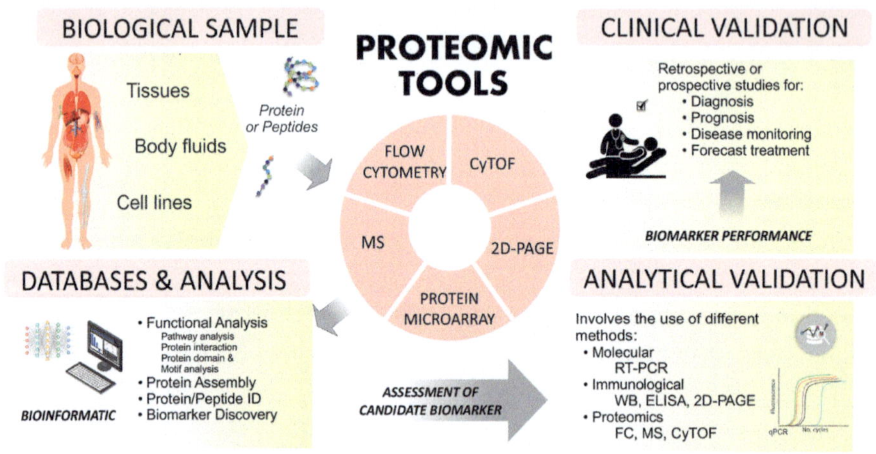

Figure 7.1: Proteomic tools as powerful approach in the investigation of BCP-ALL and the discovery of new molecular biomarkers.

Source: Proteomic tools and new insights for the study of B-cell precursor acute lymphoblastic leukemia - Scientific Figure on ResearchGate. Available from: https://www.researchgate.net/figure/Proteomic-tools-as-powerful-approach-in-the-investigation-of-BCP-ALL-and-the-discovery-of_fig1_335791502 [accessed 28 Nov 2022]

Instead of having a linear sequence, polypeptides have a tertiary structure, which reveals their three-dimensional structure. This structure is more important than the linear sequence. When referring to such a configuration, the term "tertiary structure" is typically employed. Ionic contacts, hydrogen bonds, hydrophobic forces, and van der Waals forces between R-groups are all contributors to the creation of this structure. Hydrogen bonds are also important. At this point in the hierarchy of the organizational structure, themes, and domains become more obvious. Instances of this type of pattern include the beta-alpha-beta motif, the Greek Key motif, and the Hairpin Beta-motif, amongst other examples. Modularity is one of the characteristics of the tertiary structural level, which also includes domains as one of its characteristics. Domains are sections of polypeptide chains that each include more than 200 amino acids and have the ability to fold into two or more tightly packed globular clusters. Domains can also contain several subdomains. Domains can be classified in several different ways, including alpha, beta, and mixed-beta. Proteins that include a large number of polypeptide chains have quaternary structures that are analogous to those of hemoglobin (Jones, 2013) For example, type 1 proteins are alpha proteins, which are one of four types determined by the structural characteristics that they share. You may get it in beta, as part of a package, or on its own (predominantly or core, primarily beta-strand). The following is an illustration of what an alpha/beta structure, which is typically made up of alternating alpha-helix and beta-stand structures, looks like: a rolled-up single sheet of sandwich paper that has been wrapped around the outside of a barrel. The structure known more generally as alpha beta has several distinct variations, including the pattern known as beta alpha and beta. One of the characteristics of an antiparallel beta-sheet is that its orientation is distinct from that of its neighbors.

Proteins are extraordinarily complicated molecules that are necessary for the survival of every living thing. The vast majority of proteins exist in the form of linear polymers, and each protein can be broken down into as many as 20 distinct sequences of L-amino acids. Because of their unique structures and amounts, the proteins found in a cell each play a specific purpose and have their identities. Proteins not only act as unique identifiers for the different ecotypes of microorganisms, but they are also essential for determining the energetic metabolism of every living cell. Proteins are essential for defining the energetic metabolism of every living cell. The proteomes of particular cells can provide insight into the possible distinctive qualities that each cell possesses. Proteins are engaged in a wide range of processes, ranging from the progression of diseases to the communication between cells, and each protein serves a distinct function in these processes. Because of their one-of-a-kind three-dimensional structure and the fact that they can react in response to the presence of a certain cell, proteins are great raw materials for nanofabrication. Knowledge of the three-dimensional structure of the protein is required to have an understanding of the living agent or agents that operate as toxins in a particular illness. Molecular diagnostics, which is founded on protein docking research, has made it possible to produce widely available technology that can diagnose viral diseases and infections like SARS-CoV-2 (Jones, 2013). This technology was previously unavailable. Protein docking offers an exceptionally sensitive detection method, opening up a new line of inquiry that has the potential to develop nano biosensor technology. In recent years, because of developments in nanotechnology, a new subfield of medicine known as nanomedicine has developed as a subject of research. In this field, biology, electronics, and physics are all intertwined with one another. It takes into consideration the most recent breakthroughs in regenerative medicine, diagnostic equipment, molecular imaging, and drug delivery technology. Utilizing cutting-edge sensing, processing, and operating capabilities, nanomedicine offers non-invasive diagnostics both *in vitro* and *in vivo*, as well as personalized treatments. This comes as a nice surprise, which is an added perk. Imaging systems that are powered by nanotechnology are becoming an increasingly common component of non-invasive diagnostic treatments. Examples of nanodiagnostic technology include biochips, microarrays, nanoparticle-based immunoassays, nanoscale imaging, nanoparticle-based bio labels, and a multitude of additional diagnostic instruments. These days, there is a wide range of research approaches that may be used to investigate protein-protein interactions. Each of these methodologies has its own set of benefits and drawbacks. A high level of specificity suggests that most of the identified interactions take place in the physical world, but a high level of sensitivity indicates that the majority of these interactions were recorded by the screen. Nano biosensors that are based on proteins are gaining more and more popularity for application in medical diagnostics as well as in other fields like the analysis of food, the detection of bioterrorism, and the monitoring of the environment.

These biosensors can detect in real-time the presence of protein-based poisons and viruses in live organisms. Proteins are necessary for the metabolic processes of all living organisms and play a crucial role in these activities. How a particular cell reacts to the environment around it is what gives that cell its own identity (Jones, D. T. 2013).

Docking is a process that takes place when a protein attaches to a substrate or antibody. This process causes a change in the molecular mass, shape, and physicochemical properties of the protein. Various technologies, such as nanosensors, can detect these modifications as a method of unequivocally determining whether a protein is a toxin or a living thing. Docking is one method that may be used to determine whether or not a protein is hazardous. There are other methods as well. The usage of proteins that are created by living creatures, which results in conformational changes, slow docking as a result of environmental conditions, and unstable fixing as a result of protein structure, are all at the root of the problem. Because of these problems, the use of synthesized proteins has become increasingly widespread. These proteins have been painstakingly generated and optimized with the assistance of bioinformatics resources that are available online. This brief discussion will focus on the capabilities of bioinformatics tools to optimize and compute the physiochemical characteristics of proteins that have the potential to be candidates for use in nano biosensors.

7.2 SEQUENCE ANALYSIS

The phrase "sequence analysis" is used to describe the process of doing a computational study on a DNA, RNA, or peptide sequence to learn more about its properties, biological function, structure, and evolutionary history. An appreciation for the history of the data, or the many experimental approaches that led to the biological sequence, is essential for its successful analysis. Then, depending on the type of sequence being analyzed, we'll need to employ a different set of analytic techniques (genomic, transcriptomic, or proteomic). The massive quantities of data that have lately been collected on these biomolecules must first be searched for comparable sequences in the databases that preserve this information to guide experimental testing for the aim of the functional investigation. It is standard practice in bioinformatics to take advantage of the many software programs and digital resources that are currently available. After a thorough examination of the sequences of each component, the next step is to figure out how DNA, RNA, and protein sequences relate to one another and the mapping of the genome via proteins. To comprehend the effects of these interactions on an organism's growth and survival, it is vital to study the relationships between metabolites and the genes and proteins responsible for metabolic processes. This website aims to provide an introduction to sequence analysis on all three levels (DNA, RNA, and proteins), as well as metabolic pathways that show how these levels interact with one another (Lopez, 2019).

Analyzing protein sequences can reveal details about the preferred amino acid residues and the distribution of such residues across the sequences. This is crucial for gaining insight not just into the secondary and tertiary structures of proteins, but also into the functions they play in the body. Similar motifs found in different protein sequences can help researchers figure out which sections of a protein are crucial to its structure and function. Profiles will be generated using the qualities of individual amino acids and are based on the sequence of amino acids, which will be used to group amino acids that have comparable features. The quantity of information included in amino acid sequences may be used to develop sequence-based prediction systems.

Using these techniques, we can predict which amino acids a particular sequence will yield. By applying alignment methods to compare amino acid sequences, one may gain a better understanding of the existence of similar sequences and apply them as a template to predict the three-dimensional structure of proteins. Amino acid sequence comparisons can help with this. Comparing the sequences or structures of two proteins is the major method for determining their similarities and differences. Using this method, you may establish a direct link between two proteins' amino acid sequences. I am referring, of course, to the building blocks of protein—the amino acids. Two sequences can be globally aligned to see if they share the same correspondence throughout. This is the most straightforward inference to be drawn from the alignment of the two sequences. Another option for a global alignment is a local alignment. Similarity-based alignments focus solely on the parts of the proteins that share the greatest sequence. To better understand a novel or uncharacterized protein, it is standard practice to compare it to a protein whose features have been previously established by experimentation. This helps scientists infer information about the unknown proteins' structure, function, and evolutionary history. When employing this tactic, sequence searches are typically the first port of call. The similarity between two sequences is often regarded as the most reliable indication of homologous relationships. Quality sequence search techniques include BLAST (Ladunga, 2017), HMMER (Potter et al., 2018; Prakash et al., 2017), HHblits (Remmert, Biegert, Hauser, & Soding, 2011), and HHpred (Altschul et al., 2011). Researchers in the biological sciences requested these tools so that they may more easily locate the most relevant bioinformatics resources on the web. Since then, Toolkit has continued to operate as usual. The previous version was retired in favor of a newer, improved version built using modern web technologies that offer greater scalability and reliability (Alva et al., 2016; Zimmermann et al., 2018). The Toolkit now features 35 built-in and third-party tools. To do this, we employ the MSA calculators PSI-BLAST, Clustal Omega, and T-Coffee. Secondary structure estimates are calculated with Quick2D, and sequence properties are determined with PCOILS.

The role of public enterprises in the economy of a country depends basically on its economic system. Regardless of ideology and policy, however, almost every developing country has found it desirable and even necessary to establish public enterprises in order to meet, responsibly, the requirements of its development program. Currently, there is a very strong belief in many developing nations that rapid and desired patterns of economic growth cannot be achieved without resorting to the device of the public enterprise.

Throughout its life, the Toolkit has proven to be a crucial piece of machinery for the study of molecular biology. The sensitive sequence-comparison programs HHblits and HHpred are largely to blame for this. These methods can find homologous connections in a sequence that the other methods miss. Furthermore, this part of the Toolkit ensures that all of the individual tools work together seamlessly. It is possible to accomplish this by using the output from one tool as the input for another. PSI-BLAST search results might be given to Clustal to create a MSA of the identified matches, or to MMseqs2 to build a smaller set that is filtered by pairwise sequence identity. Using both of these applications, we can limit the pool of possible partners. These two instances illustrate how the results from one tool can be repurposed by a third tool.

Comparison Mode: This manner of operation of HHpred makes it possible to compare two MSAs or protein sequences. Using a protein sequence as input, the Protocol lays out the steps that must be taken to create a unique MSA of the highest possible quality. For further processing, the HHpred algorithm takes this MSA as input. Protocol 2 aims to demonstrate the use of HHpred and MODELLER to create a 3D structural model of the desired protein sequence. Protocol 3 discusses the fundamentals of using PSI-BLAST and CLANS to find distant homologs of a protein of interest and then investigate the connections between the found homologs (Lopez, R. 2019). The purpose of this may be to learn more about the protein's family tree. This may be done to clarify the homologous connections. *Prometheoarchaeum syntrophicum* strain MK-D1, the closest cultured prokaryotic relative of eukaryotes, is included because its FtsZ protein serves as a useful example of the processes described here. In most bacteria, many archaea, all chloroplasts, and some mitochondria, an enzyme called FtsZ, are responsible for the production of filaments at the site of cell division. Both of these latter organelles are good representations of endosymbiotic eukaryotic organelles. Microtubules are an essential part of the cytoskeleton, and FtsZ is linked to eukaryotic tubulins, which are polymerized to produce these structures. It has been discovered that FtsZ is present in bacteria, yeast, and plants. GTPases like FtsZ and tubulins contain a C-terminal regulatory domain and an N-terminal GTP-binding domain with a GGGTG(T/S)G motif associated with GTP binding, as described by Nogales, Downing, Amos, and Lowe. There is a GGGTG(T/S)G motif in GTPases involved in GTP binding. In terms of structure, these two GTPases are very similar.

Less than 15% of the FtsZ and tubulin sequences that have been compared to one another are nearly similar. Since this is the case, the great majority of sequence search tools fail miserably at their intended task. A lot of work has been done to understand the structure, function, and evolution of FtsZ and tubulins, and their evolutionary link has gotten a lot of attention as well (Lopez, R. 2019).

Primary Functional Units in Protein Sequence Analysis

Proteins are assembled in a sectioned, modular way, with different portions performing specialized activities. The most fundamental component of modular systems is typically referred to as the "domain" in the industry. Regrettably, experts are unable to even come to a consensus about a common definition of "domain." Biochemists and geneticists, in contrast to structural biologists, focus on the empirically verifiable activities of organisms, whereas structural biologists are more concerned with the structural independence of organisms. Evolutionary biologists focus their research on the aspects of organisms that have changed very little, if at all, during the duration of evolution. With this updated conception, structural and evolutionary variables are given more weight than before. In the structural domain, the decade of the 1960s saw the first descriptions of structures of water-soluble globular proteins that had been resolved by X-ray crystallographic techniques. Crystallography was utilized to get this level of detail.

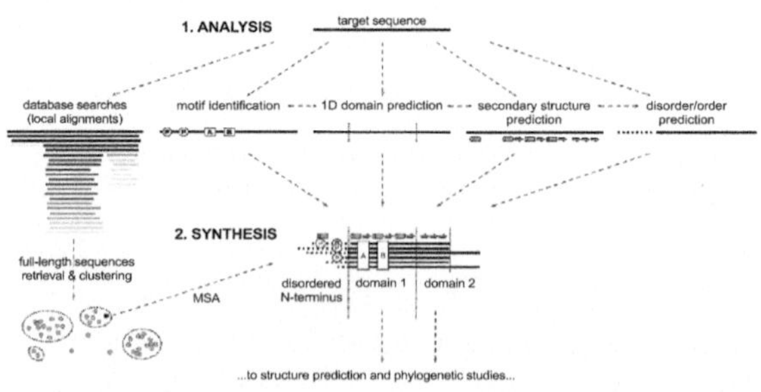

Figure 7.2: Suggested workflow for protein sequence analysis.

Source: Kaminska, Milanowska, Bujnicki, 2008. The Basics of Protein Sequence Analysis. https://doi.org/10.1002/9780470741894.ch1

The fact that the majority of globular domains have an ellipsoidal or spherical shape indicates that the internal structure of these domains is often stable. Within the structural domains of a polypeptide chain, it is possible to establish that the backbone of the chain possesses regular secondary structure (-helices and/or -strands). This three-dimensional structure, which is formed when the protein folds, acts as a scaffold for the functional side chains of amino acid residues. While certain amino acid residues form a hydrophobic core that prevents water molecules from entering the structure, others are free to interact with one another at the hydrophilic surface of the structure. This is because a hydrophobic core could be created by just a specific subset of amino acid residues. Protein domains often contain amino acid sequences that are both relatively lengthy and marked by a high degree of informational complexity. This step is conducted so that they can fulfill the earlier discussed requirements. The number of residues that make up globular domains normally ranges from fifty to three hundred, with a few significant outliers. The predominant domains in biological membranes have a geometry that is, for the most part, consistent with one another. Their hydrophobic "belt" on the exterior of their barrel-shaped bodies assures a close match with the hydrocarbon tails of the lipid bilayer by acting as a matchmaker. There is a subgroup of transmembrane proteins (TM proteins) that are made up entirely of helices; the hydrophobic core of these proteins has been replaced by an inner hydrophilic channel that is in charge of pore formation (Lopez, 2019).

Investigations that have been carried out have shown that many instances of the same structural domain can develop from inside the same polypeptide chain or in various structural circumstances. This has been proved by the studies. Comparing the sequences and structures of a vast number of proteins led to the recent discovery that structural domains are important evolutionary and functional units. This finding was made possible by the fact that structural domains are modular. Protein domains are ubiquitous in all three kingdoms of life, including the viruses that infect archaea, bacteria, and eukaryotic organisms, and this conservation extends to the proteins themselves. The helix-turn-helix domain is a frequent form of the domain that is virtually always found in proteins that bind to DNA. This is because the helix-turn-helix structure mimics the structure of DNA (Meyerson, 2012).

7.3 STRUCTURE PREDICTION OF PROTEINS

Proteins, also known as macromolecules, are vital components of practically every living thing. The process of predicting the structure of proteins mainly relies on the homology that exists between protein sequences and structures. Because the function of a protein is determined to a considerable extent by its three-dimensional structure, it is extremely important to model or predict the structure of a protein. Research into the structure of proteins is, therefore, extremely important. In a similar vein, the composition of amino acids in a protein is what determines its three-dimensional form. Even relatively little changes to the sequence of a protein can have a significant impact on the native structure of the protein. Although it is crucial to understand the 3D structure of proteins, it can be difficult to determine a protein's original form when it is placed in the physiological environment of the body. The majority of the time, X-ray crystallography and nuclear magnetic resonance spectroscopy are used to determine the structures of proteins and protein-ligand complexes (NMR). These approaches to evaluating the design of an experiment are infamous for being both expensive and time-consuming. The conceptualization of protein structure, dynamics, and folding has resulted in the development of a model that is predicated on the sequences of amino acids, in addition to a computer approach and several other computational tools (Meyerson, 2012)

Each technique, such as X-ray crystallography, nuclear magnetic resonance (NMR) spectroscopy, and electron microscopy, comes with its own set of advantages and disadvantages. In X-ray crystallography, a protein crystal is seen via the lens of an X-ray machine. The resultant diffraction pattern is recorded and analyzed with the use of computational frameworks to pinpoint the specific positions of individual atoms contained inside the molecule. This is done to determine the precise locations of individual atoms. A method known as nuclear magnetic resonance spectroscopy, or NMR for short, has shown some promise in unraveling the structural conundrum of protein-ligand complexes and other small molecules. It is possible to investigate the protein in a biologically relevant environment using nuclear magnetic resonance (NMR). There is a setting that involves water. The NMR method can only be applied to the investigation of proteins that are less than or equal to 150 amino acids in length. The use of electron microscopy allows for the creation of a tertiary model of a single particle, which may be used to study even extremely large macromolecules or even cell organelles (Cheng, 2015).

Since the beginning of time, one of the most important problems that have persisted unresolved is how a single amino acid sequence may fold into a three-dimensional (3D) protein. This is one of the most fundamental topics that has been left unaddressed. This issue has persisted for a very considerable amount of time. Analyzing protein sequences and structural data from known and validated structures has allowed researchers to investigate a wide variety of challenges associated with the packing of sequences into 3D protein models. Some of these challenges involve side chains, conformations, and helix/sheet/coil/conformations. This category contains issues related to the side chain as well as confirmations and other structural challenges. Based on these statistics and ideas, a variety of fresh approaches have been developed for the prediction of the evolution and structure of molecular molecules (Hermoso Pulido, 2015). When trying to create predictions regarding tertiary structures, one might employ a wide number of different methodologies. This is the category that contains the practices of homology modeling, threading/fold identification, and the ab initio technique.

The most significant challenge still facing structural biology is that of protein structure prediction. This endeavor is classified as NP-hard because of the extensiveness of the search space and the intricacy of the fitness landscape. There is no way to find a solution to this issue, not even with the most cutting-edge computational tools and optimization methodologies. Because there are so many instances of local minima, common approaches such as Rosetta are required to generate an extremely large number of protein models. In this scenario, and especially with the democratization of parallel computer systems, population-based meta-heuristics, like evolutionary algorithms, provide an interesting option. This is because these types of meta-heuristics are based on the idea that populations of individuals interact with one another. This holds more water than ever before in light of the way things are currently transpiring in the world. It is feasible that by employing tactics that are based on huge groups of individuals, there will be ways to spread the data.

The ability to direct the search based on information obtained from previously discovered solutions is one of the potential benefits of this feature. Other possible advantages include enhanced search space exploration as a result of a more diversified population (Meyerson, 2012). This function makes it possible for both of those possibilities to come to fruition. Along the course of a search, there is certain to be a robust conflict between gaining knowledge of the search field and making use of efficient solutions. A shift in the balance between exploitation and exploration can be brought about by adjusting and customizing population-based strategies. The factors that determine the appropriate balance vary from job to task, and increasing the effectiveness of algorithms usually necessitates the use of specialized knowledge. It is feasible to make substantial changes to the population replacement process, the solution selection, the stochastic operator choices, and even the population size while working with evolutionary algorithms. Proteins contain a wide variety of features, and there is a plethora of data that may be utilized to make it simpler for population-based algorithms to solve the challenge of predicting protein structures. These capabilities and this information can be put to use in a variety of contexts. The Rosetta engine serves as the foundation for the distribution estimation approach known as EdaRose. It has been revised to incorporate new understandings of protein structure that have been obtained via the use of computer modeling. Numerous studies have shown that population-based techniques are superior to traditional, isolated solution approaches. These strategies are more effective overall.

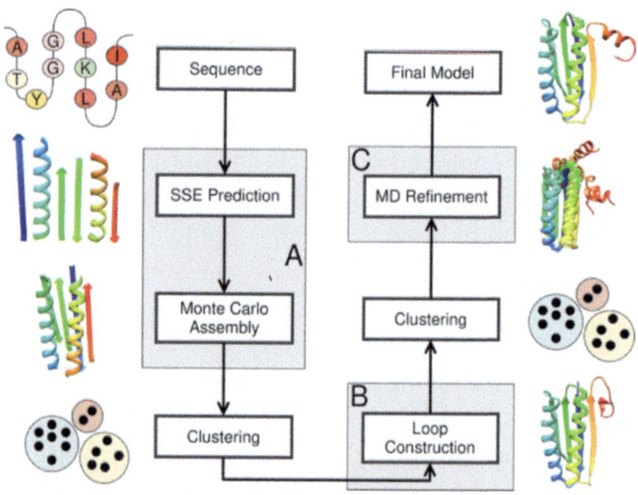

Figure 7.3: Protein structure prediction pipeline. The protein structure prediction pipeline employed in this study consisted of three modules–low-resolution topology search (A), high-resolution refinement and loop construction (B), and MD refinement (C). (A) The low-resolution topology search is based on BCL::Fold and uses machine learning algorithms to predict the secondary structure elements (SSEs) of the protein, which are subsequently arranged in the three-dimensional space using a Monte Carlo Metropolis algorithm. (B) High-resolution refinement and loop construction takes place using Rosetta's cyclic coordinate descent algorithm, followed by model relaxation. (C) Molecular dynamics simulations were conducted using the Amber package.

Source: CASP11 - An Evaluation of a Modular BCL: Fold-Based Protein Structure Prediction Pipeline - Scientific Figure on ResearchGate. Available from:

https://www.researchgate.net/figure/Protein-structure-prediction-pipeline-The-protein-structure-prediction-pipeline-employed_fig9_299769531 [accessed 28 Nov 2022]

Energy Minimization-Based Methods

When a query protein's sequence is comparable to that of another protein whose atomic structure is already known, homology modeling is the most accurate way for predicting a protein's tertiary structure. Homology modeling is the best method. This is because, during the homology modeling process, the atomic structures of both proteins are compared and utilized as reference points.

These techniques are predicated on the hypothesis that in biological systems, structures are more reliably preserved than sequences. This indicates that it is possible to build an accurate molecular model of a protein by first assigning a conformation based on sequence alignment, then creating a model, and finally minimizing the amount of energy required for the process. In other words, the process works like this: first, a conformation is assigned based on sequence alignment.

Since the sequence of the human genome is now available to the public, there has been an exponential increase in both the number of protein sequences and the distance between those sequences and the structures to which they are linked. This increase in both aspects of the problem is due to the availability of the genome sequence. As a result of this, the construction of protein models is an approach that is now enjoying widespread usage.

Creating a structure-based alignment between the query protein and a sequence for which the 3D structure is known is the first stage in homology modeling. This phase is considered to be the most important step in the process. Using this alignment, the sequence of the query protein is compared to the sequence of another protein whose three-dimensional structure is known.

When there is minimal homology between two sets of data (less than 20% of atoms in each pair are identical), the quality of perfect alignments obtained using automated methods is generally substandard.

This is because automated methods rely on computer algorithms. The geometry of the distances involved can dictate which mental angles are available for approaching homology modeling. These conceptual angles can vary greatly. This viewpoint's distance constraints, which are generated from tertiary templates, can be of use to the study of distance geometry. Modeling approaches based on homology but don't include such structures don't work very well (Meyerson, 2012).

The Hierarchical Structure of Proteins

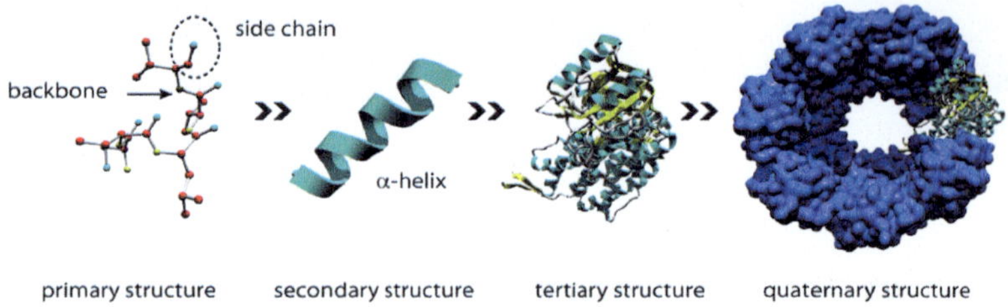

Figure 7.4: The hierarchical structure of proteins. The primary structure is defined by the sequence of amino acid residues and is responsible for subsequent folding processes. The secondary structure describes local conformations, e.g., alpha-helices or beta-sheets. The spatial three-dimensional arrangement of an individual protein is its tertiary structure. Several proteins can interact to form quaternary structures (functional multimers).

Source: Hierarchical structures made of proteins. The complex architecture of spider webs and their constituent silk proteins - Scientific Figure on ResearchGate. Available from: https://www.researchgate.net/figure/The-hierarchical-structure-of-proteins-The-primary-structure-is-defined-by-the-sequence_fig1_236237111 [accessed 28 Nov 2022]

One more method for deducing protein structures from amino acid sequences is to make use of the protein structure hierarchy. This method divides protein structures into three levels: primary, secondary, and tertiary. To understand how the sequence of amino acids relates to the tertiary structure of the protein, one must first have an understanding of how to predict an intermediate state, such as the secondary structure of the protein. A model of the protein's secondary structure is constructed with the help of the information that is included in the amino acid sequence of the protein. If one were to make use of the model provided by the secondary structure, then one might be able to predict the tertiary structure. The process of mimicking secondary proteins has given rise to several diverse methodologies. Statistical methods, physiochemical approaches, artificial intelligence-based approaches, evolutionary information methodologies, and combinatorial approaches are the five distinct methods that are currently available for researchers to select from. Unfortunately, sequencing data can only reliably predict around 80 percent of secondary structures. To apply secondary structure models to the difficult problem of predicting tertiary structures, researchers have looked into forecasting tight turns and super secondary structures in addition to the more common helices, turns, sheets, and strands. This is done to meet the challenge of predicting tertiary structures. A significant issue that has to be addressed in the field of protein structure prediction is the efficiency of the methods that are currently in use. To establish a wide array of techniques, several protein sets and evaluation criteria were utilized. The Critical Assessment of Techniques for Protein Structure Prediction (CASP) project was first conceived in 1994 as a global, open experiment to assist both inventors and customers in the protein structure prediction industry. Research conducted by CASP has the overarching goal of assessing the present state of the art in protein structure prediction. Specifically, this entails figuring out where future efforts may be most effectively focused, as well as what kind of progress has already been accomplished. The sixth version of the CASP was made available for download in December 2004. These occurrences have a frequency of once every two years on average. Other projects, such as the Critical Assessment of Fully Automatic Structure Prediction Servers (CAFASP) and the Evaluation of Automatic Protein Structure Predictions, have been formed to evaluate the efficiency of various structure prediction systems (EVA). The results of these studies will allow live web servers to be evaluated for their ability to predict protein structures.

The BLAST Sequence Analysis Tool

When a nucleotide or protein sequence is entered into the textbox on any of the BLAST websites, and the appropriate degree of coverage is selected, the website will return results from all of the publicly available sequence databases. The query is then transmitted over the Internet to the NCBI databases and servers, which search, and the results are then delivered to the user's browser in the display format that the user has selected. However, many businesses in the biotechnology sector, genetic researchers, and professionals in bioinformatics may decide to use "stand-alone" BLAST to query their local databases or adapt BLAST in some other way to make it more suitable for their specific requirements. Users of BLAST's stand-alone version have access to both the command-line executables as well as the Stand-alone BLAST Server. Customers can store confidential copies of the BLAST Web pages on their servers by utilizing the Stand-alone BLAST

Server. Comparing sequences from different kinds of databases, such as DNA databases, protein databases, and databases that include translated DNA from all six reading frames, is possible with the help of BLAST. Both PSI-BLAST and RPS-BLAST can match sequences to profiles, which is a comparable function. The score matrix provided by PSI-position-specific BLAST comes in helpful when doing repeated searches for protein sequences with similar characteristics. It does the same actions as RPS-BLAST does. After providing a quick overview of BLAST and the NCBI website, the next section will continue to cover the various BLAST outputs. The conventional report is the most well-known of these outputs; it is the default format that can be viewed on BLAST websites and goes by the name of that report type. When getting BLAST results, users have the option of selecting between pre-defined output formats or conventional reports. A hit table, XML, and ASN.1 are a few examples of formats that fall into this category. The application will make an automated decision regarding the format of the output. This chapter comes to a close with an examination of stand-alone BLAST and the numerous configuration choices it offers. The majority of BLAST's application programming interfaces (APIs) are underutilized by customers, even though these APIs might provide the key to designing applications that are more dependable and efficient. To complete the search in a shorter period, the BLAST algorithm, which is heuristic software, makes use of a wide number of innovative and effective shortcuts. The BLAST tool may be used to perform local alignments of sequences. The structure of the vast majority of proteins may be described as modular, and it is not unusual to come across functional domains that are conserved either within or between species. A modified version of the BLAST algorithm is being used to locate these areas, as well as more compact ones that contain a similar sequence. The local alignment method, which is often necessary for genome assembly and analysis, enables mRNA to be matched up with a section of genomic DNA for pairing. If BLAST were to attempt to match two sequences throughout their whole lengths, it would find fewer instances of similarity. This is especially true when considering domains and motifs (a process known as global alignment). The algorithm that runs the BLAST server retrieves the sequence together with any extra input parameters, such as the database that is going to be searched, the word size, and the anticipated result when a query is made to one of the BLAST Web sites. Creating a lookup database of all the "words" (short subsequences; for proteins, the default is three letters) and "neighboring words," or words that are similar to one another, in the query sequence is the first stage in the BLAST algorithm.

This database contains the words that make up the query sequence, which is a list of those words. The next thing that has to be done is a search inside the sequencing database to find these possible "hot spots." As soon as a match is discovered, it is immediately incorporated into the technique that is used to initiate gap-free as well as gapped expansions of the "word." BLAST does not directly scan the flat files that are stored in GenBank (or any subset of GenBank flat files). Instead, people give sequences to BLAST databases. There are two files corresponding to each entry, the first of which contains the header information and the second of which contains the sequence data. This information will be taken into consideration by the algorithm. When operating in "stand-alone" mode, the data file can be made up of either information that has been privately stored or databases from NCBI BLAST that are open to the public and have been downloaded to the local workstation. This method searches the query sequence for prospective "words" and then expands each one to its maximum length. This produces the optimal alignment for each query-sequence combination, which is then saved in the SeqAlign data structure. In addition, using this method will result in the generation of the optimal alignment for each query-sequence pair. The SeqAlign structure just refers to BLASTable sequences in place of real sequence information (Valentin, 2010).

CHAPTER 8

BIOINFORMATICS DATABASES AND TOOLS FOR WHOLE GENOME ANALYSIS

CONTENTS

8.1. INTRODUCTION

The field of bioinformatics is a branch of computer science or rather computational biology that involves the application of algorithms to biological data. This field has become increasingly important as researchers increasingly seek to understand the molecular basis of disease and to build models for disease. In itself, bioinformatics is applied in various fields, including biotechnology, molecular biology, epidemiology, evolutionary biology, and medicine. This concept can also be used to help predict how drugs will work on a specific organism or disease-causing agent. In addition to these uses, bioinformatics has been applied in many different research areas involving genetics and evolution (e.g., population genetics).

Bioinformatics can also be used to gain a better understanding of how genes function in cells. The development of new tools for bioinformatics requires access to large amounts of data. The ability to store this data in a reliable way is critical for researchers who do not have access to large computers or supercomputers. The creation and maintenance of databases searchable by key words or phrases is a powerful tool for finding information quickly and easily. Whole genome analysis is the process of analyzing a complete DNA sequence to determine its structure and function. Whole genome sequencing is an accurate sequencing technique for determining the entire DNA sequence in a sample. The whole genome sequence can be used to identify genes and their associated proteins, determine genetic disorders, predict drug targets, find new medicines, study evolutionary relationships between organisms, and much more.

8.2. THE CONCEPT OF DATA STORAGE

Data storage can be done at different levels, starting from simple storage of the raw data to complex algorithms that keep track of all the possible relationships between different data points. The hierarchy of these levels is:

- Storage of Raw data: The raw data are stored at the lowest level of data storage in whole genome analysis. This is the case when there is no other way to store the raw data, and it is the only way to ensure that the raw data is protected from any manipulation or loss. The raw data storage is also performed in four levels (Noh, T. W. 2012)

a. Raw data: This first level only relays information about the genome.

b. Raw data with coordinates for each base pair for each chromosome (BAM file format) : These BAM files contain a lot of information about the genome, but they are not easily accessible through traditional bioinformatics databases. This is because the raw data needs to be processed before it can be used in a database. The BAM files are usually stored in a database, such as GATK, which can then be used by tools to perform analysis. The GATK databases also have three levels of storage: raw, intermediate, and final. Raw data are the original files that were generated by the software to be analyzed. Intermediate files are created from the raw data when they are processed by the software. Final files are created when all other processing steps have been applied, and they are ready to be published or archived.

c. Raw data with coordinates for each base pair for each chromosome (this is called GFF file format) : Here, the raw data is stored in databases and accessed by scientists using a variety of tools. The GFF format is used to store raw data, such as DNA sequences or proteins. It contains information about the position of each base pair along a chromosome, as well as other details about the chromosome itself.

d. Raw data with coordinates for each base pair for each chromosome (this is called FASTA file format) : Data in this format can be used to perform whole genome analyses. The data is stored in a database based on the NCBI sequence file format, which can be used to store any type of nucleotide sequence. This type of data is raw and unprocessed. The name comes from FASTA, which stands for "Fasta", an abbreviation for "Fasta sequence assembly". A FASTA is a text file that lists the nucleotide sequence of each base pair in a chromosome (in this case, the human genome) with its coordinates. A FASTA can be split into smaller files known as FASTQ files or SAM files. These are ASCII files that contain compressed versions of the raw data in the original FASTA format. They are not just smaller versions of the same thing; they are different formats that allow for significant compression and easier transfer between programs and systems.

- Storage of aligned data: The alignment of the DNA sequences helps researchers better understand how genes work. The aligned data have to be stored as a level of data storage in whole genome analysis. Here, the database stores all the data from the reference genome, which is used to create a map of the entire genome.

The database also stores information about how the map was constructed and what areas need to be analyzed next. This data is the output of a read aligner, such as BWA, which maps the reads to a reference genome. The aligned data is typically stored in a SAM or BAM file, which is a compressed binary version of the SAM format (Noh, 2012).

- Storage of variant data: There are a number of different approaches that can be used when analyzing whole genomes; some of which require storing all variant data together in one place, whereas others allow for each variant to be stored separately on different databases. The data storage for variant data can be done at the level of the individual variant or at the level of the entire genome. In whole genome analysis, the variant data is stored in a database as a combination of its identity and location, allowing for easy access and search through all records.

  Variant data is typically stored as a VCF file, which is a text file containing all the variants detected by GATK or another variant caller. Whole genome analysis works by comparing the DNA of one individual to that of another to identify DNA segments inherited from a common ancestor. The output of this analysis is called whole genome variant data (WGV). It includes SNPs, indels, and other mutations in the DNA sequence. WGV is typically stored in VCF format.
- Storage of annotation data: The data gathered from WGA can be used to study the genetic make-up of an organism, its evolutionary history, or even the evolutionary relationships between different species. One important aspect of this type of analysis is the storage and retrieval of data in databases. In whole genome analysis, it is not just about storing the raw data; it is also about storing annotation data and other types of information, such as visualizations and plots. This type of storage is often referred to as "structured" storage because it follows a standard format for storing information (e.g., in database tables). It is important to note that there are different levels at which we can store our annotation data (e.g., level 1: gene sequences; level 2: exons; level 3: transcripts).

  The annotation data provides information about the genes, transcripts, and proteins that are present in the genome of an organism. The annotation data can be used to infer relationships between genes and determine how they function within an organism. These annotations also allow researchers to identify regions of interest in the genome, which can then be studied using other techniques.

Annotated data can easily be stored in relational databases. It stores many different tables or schemas that represent various aspects of your organization's data. You can create new tables and fields within each table as needed, but you must also define relationships between tables so that everything fits together properly within your system. In addition to storing your own data, relational databases also support external input from other systems like web services or APIs.

This data is the output of an annotation tool, such as Ensembl, which adds information about the functional consequences of variants. The annotation data is typically stored in a JSON or XML file. They will also store gene expression and pathway data, which can be used by downstream applications (Noh, 2012).

8.3. APPROACHES FOR THE STORAGE OF DATA USING BIOINFORMATICS-BASED DATABASES

There are three primary approaches to the storage of data in bioinformatics databases.

- Hierarchical

The first approach for the storage of data using bioinformatics-based databases is a hierarchical. In this approach, data can be stored in a hierarchical format, where each level of the hierarchy is a separate database, and each database contains related records. These systems are composed of many parts, or nodes, which are connected to each other by a number of links. In a hierarchical database, each node may have a number of children nodes connected to it by links. The parent node is always at the top of the tree and has no children nodes. The children nodes can be linked to other nodes in the database either directly or indirectly through an intermediary node called a parent node (Scheuermann, 2012).

Format

- The first step of this approach is to store the data in a hierarchical fashion; for example, you might store a list of names and their corresponding locations on a map. This is done so that if you need to find something later on, you don't have to scan through all the same information again.

- The second step is to create relationships between different types of information. For example, if you have a list of people who live in New York City, then it would make sense to link those two lists together with one another—that way, if someone ever needs to know who lives in New York City, they can easily see that information right there at their fingertips.
- The third and final step is to add additional information to the data as needed. This might include adding comments or notes about each person on the list or adding new fields such as phone numbers or addresses. By doing this, you can ensure that your data is always up-to-date and accurate, and that it can be easily expanded upon in the future.

Advantages of This Approach

The advantage of this approach is that it allows for an easy way to find specific data, such as by searching for surnames or spelling variations. It allows the user to create an organization structure that makes sense to them and their needs.

It is also quite effective in the case of data management. It would also reduce the amount of time needed to search through all your records.

Disadvantages

However, it also has its drawbacks: because each database includes only records pertaining to its own particular level, it would be difficult to link records across different levels if they did not have common fields (such as birth year). Another disadvantage is that hierarchical databases tend not to scale well when they are dealing with large amounts of data. You might be able to store billions of rows in a single branch, but if you need more space for new records, those old ones will have to go somewhere else on your hard drive or into memory while they wait their turn (Scheuermann, 2012).

- Relational approach

This approach is also similar to the Hierarchical approach. It uses the hierarchical nature of a relational database. This approach is often used with relational databases because it is easier to query and manage data using a relational schema, which allows for efficient retrieval of information based on specific criteria. The basic approach involves creating tables with columns and rows, which define relationships between data points. A table's rows represent entities like people, places, or products; columns represent attributes like names or addresses. The rows and columns are then joined together using an equality operator (such as =) to create more complex relationships between entities in your database.

Format

This approach works mainly with the use of rows and tables. Each row in the table represents a single record, and each column represents an attribute of that record. Each row has a unique primary key (also known as a unique identifier), which uniquely identifies that record. In a relational database, all rows can be accessed by their primary key. All columns in the table must have an identity value (or reference) to make them equivalent to rows in the table. For example, if there are three columns: A, B, and C, then each column must have an identity value (or reference) such as A1 or B1 or C1. This ensures that each row in the table matches exactly one column from its respective table (Noddings, 2013). For example, one table might have three fields—name, age, and gender. Another table may have six fields—username, password, email address, first name, last name, and phone number. Each record in a table has a primary key field (also called an auto-incrementing field) that uniquely identifies each row in that table. Addition of a new record to a relational database requires creating a new table with all of the same columns as the existing table; then, you can insert new rows into the new table by writing code that uses those columns to retrieve values from the existing table and create new onesentry_id = 1; In this case, entry id is the primary key for this table because it identifies each row by its column values: 1 for username and password; 2 for email address; 3 for first name; 4 for last name; 5 for phone number.

Advantages of Relational Database

The relational approach to the storage of data is one of the most popular approaches in bioinformatics. The relational approach to the storage of data is typically the most straightforward and efficient. This is because it uses a single table to store all data, with each row representing an individual piece of information. This approach is often used in databases for research purposes, as it enables users to easily find relevant information without having to sift through multiple tables or columns.

Disadvantages

The downside of this approach is that it can be very difficult to scale up if you need more space or more memory on your computer. The user has to know what type of information he/she needs and then look for it in a database. In addition, the main disadvantage is that there are many different types of databases available, which makes it difficult for users to choose one that best suits their needs (Noddings, 2013).

- Object-oriented approach

The object-oriented approach is a way to store data. It is the most common method used in bioinformatics databases. The object-oriented approach uses objects to represent biological information, such as genes, proteins, and organisms. It also allows for a more uniform representation of data across different databases and applications. This approach allows you to store the data of each particular object in an easy-to-access manner. Object-oriented databases can be created using any programming language, such as Java, C++ or C#.

In these databases, the storage of data is organized into tables and columns. Each row in the table represents a single entity; each column represents a property for that entity. For example, if we were storing information about a certain type of flower (say, roses), our table might include a column for whether or not the item was red or pink. These databases are organized into rows and columns according to their properties.

Format

In order to store an object, we need the following:

- An object class (class name and subclass)
- The fields that make up an object and their types (e.g., string or integer)
- The methods that can be called on these fields

Advantages

The objects are organized in classes or groups, then stored and accessed independently. It can also be used to write code that is independent of any programming language or database system. This makes it easier to modify specific modules without having to worry about how other parts of the application work together with them.

Objects have their fields, which can contain information about them, such as type, name, and so on. It allows for efficient searching and retrieval of information based on specific criteria such as gene name or species name. A downside to this approach is that it requires a lot more memory than other approaches because each object contains all the necessary information about itself including its size (i.e., length), type (i.e., whether it is an integer or float), etc. (Noddings, N. 2013).

Disadvantages

It is important to note that object-oriented approaches are, at times, directly compared to whole genome analysis as a sequence of analysis. In the same manner, it has some disadvantages compared to whole genome analysis.

For example, the OODB can only store information about genes and proteins. This means that it cannot store other kinds of data, such as DNA sequences or RNA transcripts. In addition, the OODB does not have any facilities for storing information about the relationships between different types of data. For example, if you wanted to store information about how many times a particular gene has been transcribed within a particular cell type, you would need to create an additional table for storing this information.

The object-oriented approach is moreover of high cost and limited scalability. This approach also limits the ability to store complex objects such as functions, classes, and interfaces. In addition, it has the limitation that only one database can be created at a time, and therefore, it does not allow for parallelization (Noddings, 2013).

Whole genome sequence data can be stored in many different ways depending on its level of accuracy:

- Accurate: The most accurate type of whole genome sequence data will contain all nucleotides in each chromosome and will accurately map regions of interest that are present throughout the genome; this type of WGS studies has been used extensively by scientists throughout history such as Thomas Hunt Morgan who discovered genetic inheritance patterns by working with fruit flies.
- Semi-Accurate: This type of WGS has less than 100% accuracy but still contains enough information about specific regions or areas within chromosomes or entire genomes that they can be used for some types of research, such as identifying genes that may play roles in disease development.

- Incomplete: This type of WGS is the least accurate and only contains limited information about specific regions or areas within chromosomes or genomes; this data is typically not useful for scientific research.

In order to create effective databases, it is necessary to first understand what you want your database to contain - what type of information should it contain? What type of format should it be stored in? Should there be any sort of structure? What types of additional information might be useful? These questions need answering before you can actually start building your database.

The following are the steps involved in preparing bioinformatics-based databases and the tools for whole genome analysis

1. Acquiring the genome sequence data from a variety of sources

The first step in preparing a bioinformatics-based database is to obtain the genome sequence data. These can come from both public and private databases, as well as experimental data generated by scientists. The data can be obtained from other laboratories that have already completed their analysis on the same organisms, or it may be given to you directly from the different authors or institutions that contributed to the study. Scientists also consider using an automated tool that searches through databases and matches the sequences against known genes. This will save valuable time by not having to manually go through each database and search for every gene.

Once you have obtained this information, you will need to make sure that all of your analyses are consistent. For example, if you have obtained sequence data for one organism, then it would not be appropriate for you also to analyze a different organism using the same software. It is also important that all of your analyses are performed using exactly the same parameters or settings (if applicable).

2. Process and format the data for analysis

   In the process of formatting, you will want to make sure that all of your data is compatible with the tools used to analyze it. If not, you will need to reformat your data before continuing with the rest of this process. Once your data has been formatted, you can begin importing it into databases such as GenBank or NCBI's BioProject database. These sites allow users to search through their databases by entering specific terms related to the specific organism being analyzed. This helps ensure that all relevant information is found and can be used for further analysis.

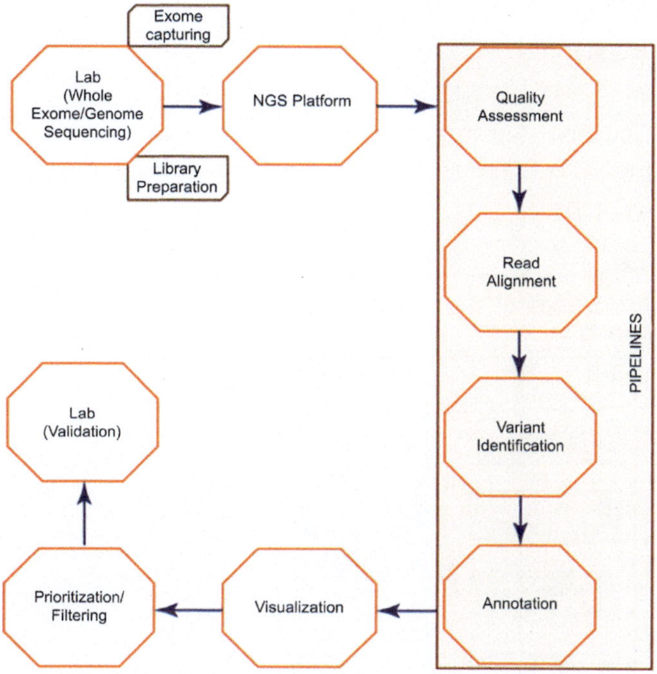

Figure 8.1: Process of preparing a bioinformatics database.

Source: Rawal, Panwar, Ali, 2017. Bioinformatics Databases: Implications in Human Health. In: Rawal, L., Ali, S. (eds) Genome Analysis and Human Health. Springer, Singapore. https://doi.org/10.1007/978-981-10-4298-0_6

Once your data has been imported into these databases, you can begin performing analysis using tools such as BLASTZ or BWA. These tools are designed specifically for use with whole genome analysis so that they can quickly identify what genes within these organisms are present or not present to determine whether or not there are any potential mutations present within them (which could be indicative of disease).

The data for analysis should be prepared in a way that allows for easy manipulation, interpretation, and analysis. The data should be stored in a format that makes it ready for further processing. It is recommended to store the data in an organized manner so that it can be easily accessed by the team members. The data should be stored in a structured way so that it can be easily accessed by the team members. This includes storing it in an organized manner with proper naming conventions and metadata tags. This helps to ensure that all information related to the study is easily accessible.

1. Storage of the data in a database

This third step involves the creation of a database, which is to be done sequentially.

- The first step in preparing a bioinformatics-based database and the tools for whole genome analysis is the storage of the data in a database.

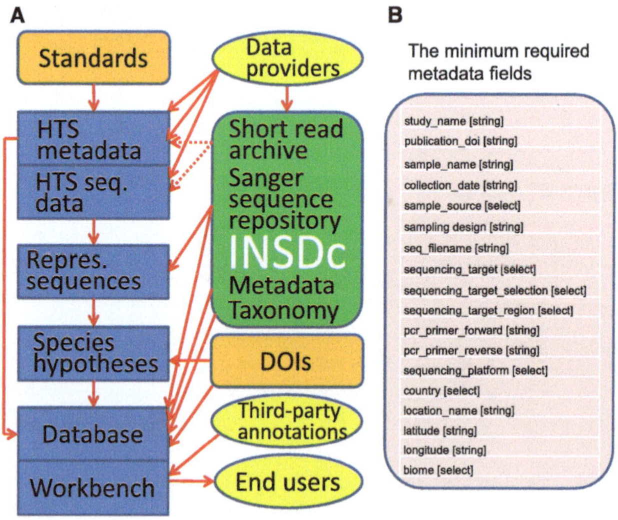

Figure 8.2: General data structure. a Suggested workflow using various bioinformatics tools and databases. DOI, digital object identifier; HTS, high-throughput sequencing; INSDc, International Nucleotide Sequence Database Collaboration; repres, representative; seq, sequencing. b Proposed minimum data fields for HTS metadata.

Source: Standardizing metadata and taxonomic identification in metabarcoding studies - Scientific Figure on ResearchGate. Available from: https://www.researchgate.net/figure/General-data-structure-a-Suggested-workflow-using-various-bioinformatics-tools-and_fig2_280629223 [accessed 28 Nov 2022]

- Next, it is important to define the types of information that will be stored in the database. This can be done by identifying the primary and secondary sources of data, as well as other relevant information such as processing instructions, formats, and other metadata that may need to be included.
- After defining the types of information that will be stored in the database, it is time to create an indexing system for all relevant

files within it so that they can be easily accessed later on by both humans and computers alike. This can be done by using either simple text-based indexes or more complex ones, depending on what needs to be done with regards to searching through large amounts of information stored within databases such as these ones!

- Another important part of preparing your bioinformatics-based database and tools for whole genome analysis involves preparing scripts that allow users to perform different operations on specific pieces of data stored within them (e.g., filtering)

Securing the data in the database is also crucial. This means ensuring that you have tight security measures in place to protect your data from unauthorized access or modification by other users. You should also consider whether or not this is something that will be done by third-party contractors or employees at your company. If you're going to outsource this work, make sure that they have access to the same level of security as you do on their part—this helps ensure that your data stays safe if someone else needs access to it. Next, you need to create a user interface for users who will be accessing the data from outside your organization's firewall or firewall rule set—this could include anyone who may want access but isn't currently part of your company's staff or security team (i.e., researchers) (Noddings, 2013).

2. Use of bioinformatics tools to analyze data.

Bioinformatics tools can be used to analyze the data. These tools are available on many different platforms, and they allow users to access a variety of resources. The first step is to prepare the database by cleaning it up, deleting any samples that are not relevant, and filtering out any duplicate entries. Next, the user will need to find all the gene sequences that were found in the dataset and create a table for each sequence. The table should include information about where the gene was located on the chromosome, what type of sequence it was (e.g., exon or intron), how many bases there were in each segment of DNA, and how long each segment was relative to all other segments in that same gene family (i.e., whether it was short or long).

These tools range from simple tools like spreadsheets to high-performance computing (HPC) systems. They work by comparing sets of similar or identical DNA sequences in different samples, which allows scientists to identify specific regions of interest within their genome. They also help researchers discover new genetic markers that could lead them down new paths toward understanding disease etiology or treatment options. Some of the functions may include;

- Identification of genes - This is done by using gene prediction algorithms and manual annotation of known proteins. This process can take several months, and it is often necessary to manually annotate the genes before they can be used for further analysis.
- Organization of the genes- Once a list of genes has been created, they must be organized into groups based on common function or biological process. This can be done through clustering algorithms such as hierarchical clustering or k-means clustering.
- Conjoining references- Once these groups have been identified, they will need to be assigned an organism or group of organisms that they reference back to when performing analyses or searches within their data set. This allows researchers to determine if any differences exist between groups in regards to phenotypes such as functional characteristics and/or traits related to phenotype expression; for example, immune system development during development may differ between different species within a given taxonomic group (e.g., humans vs. mice).
- Genome comparison- Once DNA has been identified as a gene, it can be compared with other genes to determine the function of the gene. This is called functional analysis. A functional analysis involves identifying the protein products made by a particular gene and determining if those proteins have any effect on cells or on the organism's environment.

The main purpose of genome comparison is to find similarities and differences between two or more genomes. It may also involve comparing the DNA sequences from two or more organisms to determine if they are similar enough to warrant further investigation. first step in genome comparison is to remove any single-copy genes from the genome of interest, which removes the possibility of ambiguity due to the presence of repeats in the coding sequence. After this step is complete, it is possible to determine whether the two genomes are similar enough for further analysis. One useful method for doing this is to compare their consensus sequences. If these tools find sufficient similarity between the two genomes, then it can be concluded that they are likely related and belong in the same species.

If this does not occur, then one must determine whether there are any unexpected gaps in either genome that could cause problems when aligning their sequences. This can be accomplished by running BLASTN searches against both genomes individually and checking for discrepancies between them after each search.

Genome comparisons can be done in a few different ways:

- Computational tools can be used to compare whole genomes. These tools are designed to analyze large amounts of data quickly by searching for similarities between genes and other features of the genome.
- Whole-genome sequencing (WGS) allows researchers to sequence a single organism's entire genome at once instead of just a portion at a time, as with Sanger sequencing techniques. This technique has become very popular in recent years because it allows researchers to examine all parts of an organism at once and reduces overall costs due to not having to sequence each piece individually.
- Prediction of function- The function prediction process is the first step in creating a bioinformatics-based database. The goal of this step is to get all the genes in a genome mapped and to understand their functions. For example, if you have a gene that codes for a protein and you want to know what the gene does, you could perform function prediction on your genome. If the gene is highly conserved across species, it's likely that its function will be consistent across species as well. However, if there are differences in the sequence of your gene compared to another organism's version of the same gene, then that may indicate different functions for these genes.

The first step in finding the function of an RNA is to identify the region of the genome that encodes the RNA. This process often relies on computational tools to predict which regions code for protein-coding regions and which regions code for non-coding RNAs. Once these regions are identified, it's possible to use more traditional methods like structural modeling or evolutionary analysis to determine which nucleotides are likely to encode functional RNA sequences.

The most common method used in this phase is called Gene Ontology.

Gene Ontology is a system for describing genes, their functions and relationships to each other. It is used in function prediction in whole genome analysis. In the process of whole genome analysis, first the transcriptome is extracted from the cDNA library, second, the protein coding sequences are predicted by using a database containing gene models and thirdly the protein expression patterns are mapped onto these gene models. By doing this, it is possible to identify genes whose products are present in a specific tissue or cell type.

Gene Ontology (GO) is a standard formalism for defining biological terms, which has been used extensively in function prediction in whole genome analyses.

The aim of GO is to provide a standardized language for describing the molecular function and biological process of a gene. The first draft of the Gene Ontology was published in 1997, and it has been updated several times since then. The most recent version is 2.0, released in 2008. The Gene Ontology Consortium (GOC) is responsible for maintaining this database and developing new ontologies that describe molecules' functions at the level of biochemical pathways, cellular processes, and molecular networks.

3. Interpretation of the results and using the same to answer scientific questions.

The process of preparing a bioinformatics-based database is not just about collecting data, but also about interpreting it. The database must be used to answer scientific questions. This implies that bioinformatics can be used for both discovery research and hypothesis testing. In discovery research, scientists use bioinformatics to look at large databases of information about gene function or protein function. For example, they may want to look at all the genes involved in a certain process (such as signaling), and then see which genes are most important in that process. They will then use this information to find new genes or proteins that may be involved in that process. In hypothesis testing, researchers analyze large databases of information about protein function in order to see if there are any patterns or trends that would suggest how a particular protein might work.

These are some examples of bioinformatics-based databases

4. NCBI databases

NCBI databases are a great example of bioinformatics-based databases. NCBI is the National Center for Biotechnology Information, and it is responsible for this organization's databases and portals. The NCBI database contains a number of different types of information, including gene sequences, protein sequences, nucleotide sequences, and more. It is a service of the U.S. National Institutes of Health (NIH). The NCBI provides bioinformatics services for biomedical researchers and clinicians, including databases, software and tools, and resources for analyzing biological data (Eaton, 2020).

Databases supported by NCBI include:

- GenBank - a database containing over 50 million protein sequences and over 45 million nucleotide sequences, including information on gene structure, regulation, development, and evolution
- RefSeq - an online database containing all known functional sequences from genes to proteins to genes and viruses
- Entrez - an online database containing over 8.5 million Genome Entrez Gene Nucleotide Sequence Search Results (GEDNASE) entries related to human diseases and other biomedical topics
- UniProt - an online database containing over 603,000 proteins with more than 200,000 unique sequences
- dbEST - This database contains information about ESTs (expressed sequence tags) and their associated genomic sequences from a variety of organisms. ESTs are short pieces of DNA (usually several thousand nucleotides long) that code for proteins that can be used in the search for new drug targets.
- -Genome Database Project - The Genome Database Project (GDP) is a resource for the cataloging, annotation, and analysis of human genomes. It is part of the National Center for Biotechnology Information (NCBI).
- Gene Ontology Database - The Gene Ontology Database (GO) is an ontology database containing biological concepts and relationships that have been assigned semantic annotations with respect to GO Biological Processes.
- Pathogenic Bacteria Virtual Microbiome Project - The Pathogenic Bacteria Virtual Microbiome Project (PBMVP) aims at creating an online resource on pathogenic bacteria that will allow users to explore their diversity in terms of genome sequences, gene products, virulence factors, and other relevant informatics data

5. The African Genome ariation database (AfGVD)

The AfGVD is a publicly available collection of bioinformatics data on DNA variation in Africa. It enables users to access high-quality data on vertebrate, invertebrate, and plant genomes from around the African continent. The AfGVD has been designed to meet the needs of researchers who require large amounts of high-quality data on genetic variation in Africa, as well as those who wish to use this information in their research.

It was created by scientists from the University of Cape Town and the Welcome Trust Sanger Institute in order to help identify genetic variations that contribute to disease. The database contains information about 3,586 single nucleotide polymorphisms (SNPs), which are changes between different versions of a gene or chromosome. The AGV maintains records for SNPs located in regions coding for proteins, and it also includes information about non-coding SNPs, which affect how genes are expressed. The AGV's goal is to aid scientists in their research efforts by providing them with relevant information on human genetic variation.

6. The African Genebank network

The African Genebank Network (AGN) is a bioinformatics-based database that is designed to facilitate the identification and recording of genetic diversity in the African flora. The database is made up of 47,000 sequences from different taxonomic groups and provides information on their origin, occurrence, conservation status, and utility. It was founded in 1992 by the National Research Foundation of South Africa and has grown to include more than 70 countries across Africa.

The main goal of this organization is to help those who need access to these resources on the continent, as well as those who are interested in them. The organization has been working with researchers from around the world to develop new ways of using these resources for their own research purposes. They also provide training and support for local scientists who have an interest in using this information for their own work. One example of a project that involves this group is the creation of a database that lists all the plant species found in South Africa. This database will allow researchers from around the world to search through it when they need specific plants for their own studies or projects. It will also make it easier for people from South Africa who want to grow plants locally without having access to them elsewhere first (Eaton, 2020).

8.4. TOOLS FOR WHOLE GENOME ANALYSIS

These tools are dependent on the goals of the analysis e.g.

- Sequencing technologies
  - ✓ Whole genome sequencing

Whole genome sequencing is a method of analyzing the complete DNA sequence of an organism. It can be used to determine the genetic make-up of an organism, which can be useful in many fields, including medicine, agriculture, and forensics. Whole genome analysis has been used in labs around the world since 2001 and is one of the most commonly used sequencing techniques in biotechnology today.

✓ Whole exome sequencing

Whole exome sequencing is a "sequencing technology that analyzes the complete set of genes in a genome." It is the most expensive and time-consuming method of whole genome analysis. Whole exome sequencing is used to identify mutations in the protein-coding regions of DNA, which are responsible for making proteins. The process involves taking a sample of tissue and extracting RNA before sequencing it.

- Alignment algorithms

✓ Bowtie

Bowtie is a tool that aligns short DNA sequences. It was developed by frequently used in whole genome analysis. As its name suggests, it uses a bow-shaped curve to guide the search for the best alignment. Bowtie is one of the most popular methods for aligning DNA sequences, due to its high accuracy and speed. In fact, it has even been used on very large datasets with up to 10 million long reads. It can also be used in conjunction with other algorithms like MAFFT or MUSCLE. Bowtie works by breaking up the dataset into fragments of equal length and finding the best set of fragments that can be aligned together. It then uses this information to produce a bow-shaped alignment curve that shows how well each fragment aligns with its neighbors.

- Variant calling tools

✓ VarScan

VarScan is a variant calling tool that uses the Illumina HumanHap300 BeadChip to identify variants. It is designed for analysis of whole genome data, and it can be used on any software platform. The tool uses a machine learning algorithm to identify common variants and then uses the information to train a classifier for identifying variants that are not in the reference genome. It provides a detailed list of variants in your genome, including their locations and frequencies, along with information about how they may affect gene function. VarScans can be used to check for homozygous deletions, insertions or duplications, as well as single nucleotide polymorphisms (SNPs), which are changes in the DNA sequence of genes.

- Genome Analysis Toolkit (GATK)

The GATK, was developed by a team of researchers at Harvard University and is widely used today in genomics research. The tool identifies all variants in a genome by comparing the reference human genome to the DNA sample of each individual. The tool allows researchers to determine whether or not a particular variant has been seen before and also checks for duplicate reads from different sequencing platforms. The version 2.0 release of GATK includes a tool called Cufflinks that can be used for alignment-free contig assembly. This tool has been widely adopted by researchers because it does not require any manual intervention on the part of the user.

- Annotation platforms
- Ensemble

Ensembles are a type of annotation platform that uses a machine-learning algorithm to identify patterns in the genome. They are useful for looking for rare variants, which can be difficult to find without a machine-learning algorithm. It allows users to analyze millions of DNA sequences at once and compares the results of each individual sequence with the others in order to create a comprehensive picture of the genetic make-up of an organism.

- UCSC

UCSC is an annotation platform that allows users to annotate or predict gene expression from DNA, RNA and protein sequences. The UCSC Genome Browser is an online tool that can be used for searching and visualizing genomic data. The UCSC Genome Browser provides a free and open-source tool for exploring genomes. It allows users to explore genomic sequence information from all organisms and genomes, including those from bacteria, plants, animals, and humans. Using the Genomic Resources Database (GRD), the browser can be used to study the whole genome of any organism.

Users can search through gene descriptions, genes that have been annotated with functional information (such as proteins or metabolic pathways), expressed sequence tags (ESTs), and duplicated genes and genes that are not found in databases such as Entrez Gene or NCBI Entrez Protein database. They can also search by specific features, such as sequence conservation between species or between regions of homologous chromosomes in different species, using BLASTN alignment algorithms.

CHAPTER 9

MAIN CHALLENGES IN THE FIELD OF BIOINFORMATICS

CONTENTS

9.1. INTRODUCTION

Bioinformatics uses computers to acquire, store, analyze, and disseminate biological data such as DNA and amino acid sequences. Scientists and clinicians utilize biological data databases to better understand health and sickness, and in certain cases, medical therapy.

Bioinformatics is like data analysis in the Internet age. Before recently, data access was difficult. DNA decoding advances have decreased this barrier. Next comes data analysis and interpretation. Given the magnitude of web analytics or the human genome, computational techniques are preferred. Human genome-based bioinformatics research promises to shed light on human biology and health (Ghouila, 2015). Researchers have long sought to understand how science works. Population expansion has led to this ravenous appetite. From the microscope through cloning, stem cell research, AI, and the human genome project, every attempt has been made to understand life science. Recent transdisciplinary bioinformatics research has resulted in a full understanding of molecular biological processes, satisfying a human need for purity and wholeness. Bioinformatics deciphers gene sequences to shed light on biological problems such as embryogenesis, morphogenesis, development, neuron function, and behavior. Pharmaceutical, agricultural, and hybrid plant companies are all building bioinformatics divisions to find fresh targets and replace decreasing natural resources. Bioinformatics researchers developed new methods for studying DNA sequences and launching genomics. Gene biology's revolution has led to the development of lab processes and computer algorithms that can examine several genes concurrently. Gene expression research has spurred bioinformatics to build innovative analytic tools, improving gene-to-expression understanding and solving urgent challenges.

- Data deluge: The amount of data that is available for analysis is growing as a result of the continual development of high-throughput measurement methods. Each piece of biological data may be measured using any number of technical parameters, and it is not always clear which of these are important. Only after several iterations of quality control, filtering, normalization, and processing—all of which can include ad hoc cut-offs, settings, and procedures—can biological discoveries be achieved. Unless all pertinent data is retained, complete repeatability cannot be guaranteed. In addition, consideration of data processing, storage, and transmission among cooperating parties is necessary and frequently constrained.

Costs associated with data preservation may be substantial, even with sophisticated information reduction measures. How to choose which data sets to archive and which to discard was one of the main topics covered at the HUB conference. Participants recommended using a benefit-cost ratio to each dataset to help direct these decisions. The expected "scientific value" to the community, the cost of archiving, and the cost of creating a comparable data collection should all be taken into account when calculating a quantitative score of this kind. Initially, a technique for calculating the cost-benefit ratio was offered; however, it soon became clear that determining a genuinely accurate cost-benefit ratio score needed an assessment of the data set's scientific value a priori. Determining an exact definition of "scientific value" remained problematic because the formula was only offered at the end of a session, and many participants believed this element was hard to assess, subjective, and occasionally biased. Quantitative ratings should only be used to support those in charge of data management, participants at the HUB agreed. Even if data collection has little value to the community, it should be archived because it can never be replicated.

- Knowledge management: It is not enough to simply have information; it must also be usable and accessible. Its implementation is hampered by a lack of specified formats, common data interfaces, inconsistent biological entity IDs, insufficient support for data-exchange frameworks, and a lack of visibility. Numerous Ph.D. initiatives are attempting to solve this issue by developing a new, consistent norm to eliminate disparities. Unfortunately, these measures merely serve to muddle issues more until universally acknowledged standards are established.

  Accepting parallel interfaces while making fresh resources available in as many formats as possible, such as flat file download, BioMart access, and the Distributed Annotation System, might be a solution. Users can use these resources according to their preferences. Similar to systems biology, redundant data access can improve the reliability of data-driven algorithms (Ghouila, 2015).

- Predicting, not just explaining: Data-driven hypotheses, or the idea that data collection takes place before the development of a tested hypothesis, have received a lot of attention. In actuality, the idea is supported by the evidence. In this environment, HUB participants discussed tool integration, negative gold standards, and hypothesis vs. data-driven research.

During the symposium, there was a lot of discussion about whether bioinformaticians can successfully develop fresh ideas before carrying out actual work. Experimentalists frequently provide new data more quickly than bioinformaticians can formulate confident forecasts in many fields, particularly if bioinformaticians are consulted after the experiment has been finished. Historically, experimentalists were in charge of designing experiments and formulating hypotheses, with bioinformatics being seen as a post-hoc analysis stage. With the development of high-throughput methods, whose hypotheses are occasionally created post-experiment, there may be bias in the data interpretation. We thought that early project bioinformatics input might help to establish hypotheses and enable experimental design with the necessary statistical power to support or disprove the hypotheses, as well as guarantee that data interpretation bias is minimized. For an iterative cycle of hypothesis creation, data gathering, and hypothesis testing, further data exploration insights may be used to develop new hypotheses. Major systems biology initiatives like the Virtual Liver Network try this to some level. Models are built utilizing pre-existing biochemical data, hypotheses are developed based on the model, experiments are designed to test these hypotheses, and the new results are fed back into the original model in an iterative cycle. One option to improve this collaboration is to put pressure on funding organizations to encourage it during the grant-writing process or in conjunction with investments in facilities that will generate high-throughput data, which will almost likely need bioinformatics analysis.

The widespread integration of bioinformatics tools into traditional tools like molecular viewers, workflow managers, and modular pipelines could aid bioinformaticians in working more quickly and effectively in addition to the aforementioned improvements (Ghouila, 2015). The incorporation and reuse of tools inside molecular viewers, as well as the use of libraries like Open Babel, in projects requiring the reading and writing of several file formats, are proving useful, for instance, in the field of structural bioinformatics and simulation. Bioinformatics education should highlight the use of these kinds of auxiliary libraries as a first choice rather than an afterthought when creating new code to encourage the utilization of these strategies.

Participants at the symposium also stressed the need of having high-quality "negative gold standards" in several domains, such as collections of harmful protein-protein interactions, lists of proteins that are not drug-resistant, or decoys in protein or ligand docking studies. It is essential in this context to have access to high-quality data sets for fresh training approaches so that findings may be appropriately expanded to forecast future observations, as in medication development and customized medicine, for instance (Ghouila, 2015).

- Personalized medicine: As sequencing technology improves, personalized medicine will almost probably become a scientific reality, but the benefits to industry and public health from this trend have yet to be determined. Several important technical considerations, including whether to take a holistic approach by linking many causal links or a reductionist approach by targeting individual biomarkers, must be decided before applying any new technique of diagnosis. Some early HUB members pushed for more holistic approaches, while others leaned toward a more reductionist stance. A reductionist distillation of data may be necessary to use this knowledge in the clinic, although holistic techniques can be valuable for obtaining new information and understanding the behavior of a whole network or system. Our knowledge of the genetic and molecular basis for each disease led us to this conclusion. Both scenarios, however, need rigorous quality controls and gold standards to avoid any potential for bias brought about by, say, the employment of a variety of methods or sequencing platforms (Ghouila, 2015).

Participants discussed scientific questions, with some learning more about system biology approaches and others toward focusing on specific targets, as well as ethical and privacy issues related to the confidentiality of the data generated and the potential impact on the job market and insurance companies. This led to participants asking themselves, "Are the right social structures in place to provide fair access to this new treatment and to support folks dealing with such evident diagnoses?" and other pragmatic considerations. Some of these objectives include spreading accurate information and building public faith in scientific methods (Ghouila, 2015). Determine whether or not new research is funded to solve technical barriers like secure data storage by answering these crucial questions. Many countries and government organizations have started passing laws to deal with privacy issues and moral dilemmas associated with individualized medicine, which is great.

Learning the intricacies of a disease can, hopefully, result in a treatment that stops or even reverses the illness. Methodical research on the interplay of pharmaceuticals, proteins, pathways, mutations, and other molecular factors that affect human health is required. The HUBs had a generally optimistic view on these matters, and this was especially true in light of recent applications, technological breakthroughs, bioinformatics advances, and increased financial support for projects focusing on personalized health research, such as the 1000 Genomes Project, large-scale open access databases of drug side effects, high-throughput experimental data repositories, and increasingly predictive tools, such as those for treatment outcomes.

- Inferring the tree of life: Even though there are well-built algorithms available, there are no objective criteria for conducting orthology assignment, the initial step in generating a multi-gene or whole-genome multiple sequence alignment (MSA). The vast majority of respondents held the opinion that the number of universal (housekeeping/core) genes shared by the vast majority of Earth's creatures was insufficient for deducing a strong tree of life. We coined the phrase "gene sampling pyramid" to describe a strategy for using a very small number of genes to "get the entire picture." Additional genes might be utilized to determine evolutionary connections within and between different families and orders.

The ability to precisely determine orthology and resolve the problem of gene sampling necessitates a critical evaluation of several methodological issues, such as addressing lateral gene transfer, the issue of gene tree—species tree discordance, and the reconstruction accuracy per se of methods for MSA and phylogenetic inference. In addition, as a result of the data flood, the availability of resources (storage and processing power) is expected to become a bottleneck; the discipline is transitioning into "mainstream" computer science, on par with fluid dynamics and astrophysics. Even though it was raised in the context of "inferring the tree of life," the threat posed by defective code and a lack of verification in complicated and large-scale data analysis pipelines are universal to computing.

- Challenges in Developing a New Product: There are several difficulties in using biotechnologies to develop new products or change old ones. Designing and successfully manufacturing the planned product in the lab is the first level of achievement. The next stage is to produce the product on a modest scale and analyze the industrial structure statistically. The efficient manufacturing, fabrication, and intended use of the bio-modified product are prerequisites for forecasting and managing the difficulties related to biotechnology marketing.
- Challenges in Marketing a New Product: Time is the most significant impediment to developing innovative or novel goods from simple ideas. Because there are so many competitors on the market, the time it takes to verify, prototype, and develop a concept into a usable invention has a substantial impact on the product's success. The market has an impact on the product's success. The item should meet both the needs of the buyer and the technological demands of the moment. Technology serves as the foundation for developing a product. Technology skill sets determine the product's quality. The skills required to study and develop a new product are critical. Because of their expertise and practical experience, talented professionals are in high demand. Funding is vital for bringing a concept from the lab to the market. It must be included at every level of a product's development and life cycle. This, in turn, influences how quickly the items will be accessible.
- Policy challenges: Researchers are forced to construct items with high standards in each of modeling, and client needs fulfillment since the innovative product generated must compete with the expanding speed of new goods in the market. A profitable and distinctive product should be protected and managed using intellectual property rights. The idea that attracts attention and controls the market economy has, therefore, been legally claimed by the creator as the state of the art (Ghouila, 2015).

9.2. PROCESSING LARGE-SCALE ROBUST GENOMIC DATA

Microarray-based genotyping approaches, previously limited to analyzing regions of known variation, are being phased out in favor of sequencing technologies as they become more widely available and cost-effective. A whole genome or a few dozen exomes may currently be sequenced in roughly two weeks with an error rate of less than one per 100 kb. Even with such low error rates, there might be a large number of errors; for example, a 3 GB human genome would include around 30, 000 inaccurate variant calls (Huang, 2015).

Because of the high error rates of these technologies, applications such as detecting novel variants, face significant challenges. Each freshly sequenced genome should contain between 100,000 and 300,000 previously discovered SNPs, as well as about 1,000 somatic mutations every generation. The expected number of mutations may decrease as new genomes are sequenced; yet, the sheer volume of errors makes variant discovery a "needle in a haystack" difficulty. Because of this false positive rate, any novel variations detected will still need to be verified. High-throughput sequencing also makes finding other forms of variation more difficult, such as tiny insertion-deletion variants (indels), copy number variations (CNVs), and structural variants (SVs). New approaches for calling indels, CNVs, and SVs from reading data will be critical in recognizing these types of mutations in clinical applications.

Even high-quality sequence reads must be placed in their genomic context to discover differences, and this is a current area of study since, for example, alternative mapping and aligning algorithms sometimes provide conflicting results. Because de novo assembly is slow and complicated by repetitive areas, sequences are frequently mapped to a genomic reference sequence rather than being assembled from scratch. Smith-Waterman and BLAST are two regularly used methods, albeit their speed is affected by the size of the genome. While a single query on a single CPU may only take a few seconds, aligning 100 million of them would take more than three years (Huang, 2015).

New algorithms are being developed to address this issue. BLAT is similar to traditional sequence alignment; however, it uses a genome index rather than a linear search. Several programs, notably BLAST, have been optimized for quick-read alignment by applying heuristics such as prefix and suffix trees, hashing, or other approaches. BWA, used for the 1000

Genomes Project, is exceedingly precise, with 0.1% errors for simulated data, and can map around 7 GB of short reads each CPU day. This work is best performed in a cluster or cloud computing environment, which may be used for speedy computational analysis of secure healthcare data. To obtain the standard 30X coverage, 13 CPU days would still be required.

Short read assemblers are still plagued by reference sequence bias, which occurs when reads with stronger similarities to the reference sequence map are more frequent than reads with valid variances. A new study addresses the need to exercise caution in these alignments to avoid blunders. Allowing mismatches comes with a cost since the program must avoid creating spurious alignments. Reference sequence bias is critical for making heterozygous SNP calls and analyzing allele-specific expression using RNA-Seq data. Longer reads exacerbate the problem: whereas one mismatch is acceptable for 35 bp reads, it is insufficient for 100 bp reads.

When mapping RNA-Seq reads to a sequenced genome, reference sequence bias can be minimized by mapping the reads to both strands when the diploid sequence is available. As illustrated by the Marth Lab's MOSAIK system, using ambiguous base codes offers an alternative method of storing repeated sequences (Michael Stromberg, Boston University). Using this strategy, a C/T SNP may be represented as Y. Because the genome is typically stored in a hashed data structure, this form requires more storage. To accommodate the new codes, further keys and mappings are required (Huang, 2015).

Developing fresh methodologies for novel SNP identification provides another challenge, while frequent variations in a database like dbSNP can aid in the calling of those variants, detecting uncommon and novel variants will necessitate more confidence in the SNP call. Reference alignment methods are biased, while de novo alignment methods need too much calculation time to be practical. It is challenging to develop unique, computationally tractable algorithms while avoiding reference sequence bias (Huang, 2015).

Improving quality control measures is also critical. We may measure the mapping and SNP call quality by comparing the ratio of transition (purine/purine or pyrimidine/pyrimidine) to transversion (purine/pyrimidine) substitutions. These ratios (2-2.1) were determined during previous sequencing efforts, and we expect to observe them for newly found human genomes.

The rate of Mendelian inheritance error (MIE) can be used to assess defects in family-based genomes. Incorrect inheritance combinations are most usually the result of errors. The transition/transversion ratio and MIE metrics are used by most notable research, including the 1000 Genomes project, to assess the quality of datasets. To find novel variants at the individual SNP level, we must rely on relative quality evaluations, which must be independently confirmed. Variants can be validated using genotyping arrays or targeted resequencing. Another alternative is to resequencing the whole genome with orthogonal sequencing technology, which is more expensive and time-consuming (Huang, 2015).

9.3 INTERPRETATION OF THE FUNCTIONAL EFFECT AND THE IMPACT OF GENOMIC VARIATION

The functional impact and influence of genetic variations must be examined after genomic data processing. The statistical associations of SNPs with a variety of common illnesses have been assessed using genome-wide association studies (GWASs). It is challenging to comprehend the functional connection between related variations and phenotypic features, although these methodologies are producing new insights due to the tiny number of variants that have been discovered.

A single nucleotide variation with an allele frequency higher than 1% in the human population is considered an SNP in the strictest definition. In this study, the term "SNP" is used generically to refer to unusual changes that are seen in a smaller percentage of the population. For evaluating the effect of SNPs, data management, retrieval, and quality control are crucial considerations. In recent years, the number of SNPs that are known has increased exponentially. The most comprehensive collection of SNP data from diverse species may be found in the dbSNP database. The database had over 20 million validated human SNPs as of the time of publishing (Build 132, September 2010). A comprehensive collection of germline mutations in genes associated with hereditary diseases in humans is available in the Human Gene Mutation Database (HGMD). The free edition for research and non-profit users contains around 76, 000 mutations from 2900 genes. In the SwissVar database, 56, 000 carefully annotated missense SNPs (mSNPs) from more than 11, 000 genes are included.

Another significant source of SNP information is the Online Mendelian Inheritance in Man (OMIM) database of human SNPs and their relationships to Mendelian diseases. The PharmGKB database includes over 3400 annotated drug-response variants and over 40 VIPs, which are genetic variations known to affect drug response. These relationships between genes and medications have been extensively curated. The Catalogue of Somatic Mutations in Cancer (COSMIC) at the Sanger Institute has 25, 000 different somatic mutations associated with human cancer that were collected from the literature (Huang, 2015).

In recent years, several computer programs for predicting hazardous missense SNPs have been created. Among the approaches used in these methods were Empirical Rules, Hidden Markov Models, Neural Networks, Decision Trees, Random Forests, and Support Vector Machines.

Amino acid sequence, protein structure, and evolutionary data are frequently used as input features for prediction algorithms. The changed residues' physicochemical features, such as hydrophobicity, charge, polarity, and bulkiness, dictate the characteristics of the amino acid sequence. Protein structural information specifies the structural context of the mutation and has been successfully applied to forecast changes in protein stability brought on by mutation. Some of the most crucial elements for determining the impact of missense SNPs are provided by evolutionary research: Since essential amino acids are usually conserved throughout protein families, changes at conserved locations are typically detrimental.

New algorithms are being developed that use knowledge-based data. Two techniques for predicting mSNPs based on evolutionary information are SIFT and PolyPhen. While PolyPhen predicts the effects of mSNPs based on various sequence-based features and a position-specific independent counts (PSICs) matrix derived from MSA, SIFT scores the normalized probabilities for all potential substitutions based on a MSA of homolog proteins. The PANTHER technique uses a collection of protein family hidden Markov models to predict dangerous mutations. This study found that 3D structural traits improved the prediction of disease-related mSNPs. The accuracy of prediction algorithms has been raised to more than 80% using knowledge-based information. For instance, the functional information-based method SNPs&GO accepts as input log-odd scores obtained from Gene Ontology (GO) annotation terms. MutPred analyzes and predicts the likelihood of structural and function gain or loss as a result of mutations using a Random Forest-based method. More details on mSNP predictors have recently been examined, and a few methods for predicting dangerous mSNPs are presented.

Experimental testing is necessary to validate genetic predictions since prediction tools do not provide information on disease pathogenesis. There is a need for rapid and accurate methods for gene prioritization since laboratory validation is expensive and time-consuming. The notion of similarity to genes linked to the biological process of interest is presently used by the most effective approach (guilt-by-association). Functional annotation, protein-protein interaction (PPI) data, biological pathways, and literature are all used as input data in the current gene ranking methods (Huang, 2015).

The SUSPECT method chooses genes by contrasting sequencing traits, gene expression information, Interpro domains, and functional keywords. ToppGene combines human gene annotations, literature, and mouse phenotypic data. MedSim combines functional data from human disease genes or proteins and their orthologs in mice models. ENDEAVOUR assesses prospective genes based on a variety of genomic data sources and is trained on genes connected to well-known biological processes. The G2D prioritization method is based on a combination of sequencing properties and data mining from biological databases. To find connections between human diseases, genes, mutations, drugs, pathways, tissues, organs, and metabolites, PolySearch searches biological databases. By contrasting the human phenome and disease phenotypes, MimMiner employs text mining to rate phenotypes. PhenoPred uses the human PPI network, known gene-disease correlations, protein sequences, and protein functional information to uncover gene-disease linkages at the molecular level. By analyzing gene lists and choosing genes for functional testing, GeneMANIA develops gene function hypotheses. The method examines input genes from six species using data from several general and organism-specific functional genomics datasets. For further information on gene prioritizing methods, consult a recently published review and the Gene Prioritization Portal, which provide in-depth explanations of the predictors that are now in use.

The methods for SNP analysis are mostly limited to estimating the effects of missense SNPs. New methods are needed to evaluate the impact of synonymous, synonymous deletion, and insertion SNPs. To evaluate the effects of intronic SNPs, such as those located in promoter regions and splicing sites, functional parts of the genome must also be identified. Identification of conservation across species is more challenging in non-coding regions. Fortunately, our ability to predict the effects of non-coding mutations will increase as the number of functionally annotated genomes increases. Variations in regulatory areas may have functional consequences since SNPs in transcriptional motifs, for instance, might affect transcription factor binding. Recently, a method known as is-rSNP for locating possible genetic variations in regulatory regions was created. Is-rSNP uses phylogenetic data and transcription factor binding site prediction to find variations in potential cis-regulatory regions. Identifying changes that affect the splicing location is also required. Using the Skippy technique, one may predict major effects on gene function brought on by splicing disruption by looking at the genomic region surrounding the variant. The methods for identifying dangerous mutations in non-coding DNA have recently been explained in more depth.

The first Critical Assessment of Genome Interpretation (CAGI) was held last year to assess the various methods for anticipating the effects of genetic variation on phenotypes and to stimulate further investigation. In the first year, the CAGI organizers provided six unique data sets for six distinct objectives. Only two sorts of experiments were predicted by the majority of participating groups: experiments connected to sickness and trials that modified function. The following types of predictions were made by a few organizations: risky SNPs from GWAS research, analysis of Personal Genome Project data, prediction of P53 function alterations, and responsiveness of breast cancer cell lines to various therapies. For disease and functional forecasts, several established predictors performed well, while new categories showed potential. Future quality improvements brought forth by competitions like CAGI will refresh the difficulty of understanding genetic variation data (Huang, 2015).

9.4 INTEGRATING SYSTEMS AND DATA TO CAPTURE COMPLEXITY

Given the multiple phenotypes necessary in personalized treatment, the usual "one-SNP, one-phenotype" strategy utilized in most studies is insufficient. The bulk of medically relevant phenotypes is thought to be caused by gene-gene and gene-environment interactions. Medication response, for example, usually relies on many pharmacokinetic and pharmacodynamic interactions that, when combined, form a powerful and tolerant system with many diverse interaction partners and highly polymorphic enzymes. Because of its complexity, a drug-response phenotype of interest is likely to be impacted by numerous genes and environmental factors. The majority of diversity in response to warfarin has been linked to just two genes, CYP2C9 and VKORC1, suggesting low success using the standard GWAS approach for pharmacogenomics. As a result of these and other warfarin studies, an upgraded dosage algorithm that surpasses the current clinical algorithm has been established. Variations in CYP2C19 have also been connected to clopidogrel responsiveness. Despite this accomplishment, there remains a dispute on whether conventional techniques for pharmacogenomics will be helpful. Small sample sizes, selection biases for genetic variations, interactions with the environment that may alter outcome measures, and multiple gene-gene interactions that may be accountable for unexplained effects are all acknowledged drawbacks of pharmacogenomics GWAS. These constraints make it difficult to comprehend unexpected phenomena, such as the pharmacogenetics of adverse events.

Because GWAS approaches are designed for single marker correlations, they have difficulties in characterizing the heredity of sickness. When used in pharmacogenetics, these same methodologies are unlikely to perform significantly better. In practice, if these algorithms are parameterized for the multiple-marker correlations necessary for pharmacogenetics, they will suffer from the "curse of dimensionality" and lose a significant proportion of statistical power. For a genome with 1 million SNPs, for example, it would take around 500 billion possibilities to investigate all potential combinations of two SNPs. To deal with this complexity, bioinformatics must develop algorithms that combine several data sources while maintaining statistical strength.

Several groups have previously attempted to manage this degree of complexity in GWAS for sickness. Although both forward and comprehensive searches were done, the latter may have missed some associations, while the former may have lost statistical power. Model selection approaches have proved helpful in disease and trait GWAS studies by applying selection algorithms to create multifactorial models that balance the false positive rate, statistical power, and processing demands of the search (Tugwell, 2011).

Given the size of the genomic datasets, dimensionality reduction techniques like principal components analysis, information gain, and multifactor dimensionality reduction will be critical to make complexity algorithms reasonable. Some of these strategies have been successful in identifying multilocus associations with illnesses such as hypertension and familial amyloid polyneuropathy type I. A recent paper categorizes and covers various feature selection approaches for bioinformatics. These strategies can be quite effective when working with massive datasets; however, they do not involve any outside knowledge sources or explain the biology underpinning the links (Tugwell, 2011). Systems biology and network techniques address the issue of complexity by merging molecular data from several levels of biology, such as genomes, transcriptomes, metabolomes, proteomes, and functional and regulatory networks. A disease or medication response phenotype can be viewed as a disturbance in the global network from its stable state. To determine which genes or gene combinations, as well as other biological indicators, are more likely to be associated, biological knowledge from networks must be integrated.

Combining many data sources can show unexpected linkages and offer information on gene-environment interactions. One group created a disease-gene network by combining illnesses and associated genes found in OMIM. The examination of this network indicated that disease genes are commonly non-essential and are not necessarily hub genes. The same group created both a PPI network and a drug-target network. The network shows that related medications cluster together, that etiological and palliative drugs have separate topologies, and that experimental and newer pharmaceuticals tend to be polypharmacological. Chemical structure, disease indication, and protein sequence may all be used to map out the whole pharmacological space, which can subsequently be used to predict polypharmacology. Using epigenetic data may also help us better understand pharmaceutical phenotypes.

Pathway and gene set techniques can also be utilized when a group of genes in a GWAS is deemed to be connected. These approaches are equivalent to Gene Set Enrichment Analysis (GSEA) for microarray expression data. Other, more precise techniques have been devised, while a traditional statistical test is frequently used to determine if a set of genes is connected. Prioritizing Risk Pathways combines genetic and route data into a single metric, whereas the SNP Ratio Test compares the number of SNPs in a pathway to permuted sets (Tugwell, 2011).

Many organizations anticipate that the integrated systems biology method will successfully link genetic measurements with medicinal applications. One group employed PPI, pharmacogenomics interactions, and chemical similarity metrics to develop a pharmacogenetic prediction approach. Another group hypothesized and confirmed new "off-target" interactions using comparable pharmacological ligand sets.

These systems approaches are fascinating, but bioinformaticians must proceed with caution since there are a few pitfalls. Methods must be based on high-quality data to avoid the "garbage-in, garbage-out" phenomenon, especially when one inaccurate assumption might spread across several data sources and magnify the inaccuracy. Moving annotations based on similarity, for example, may occasionally work but may falsely associate a paralog with a function. When comparable molecules are chemically identical, they might behave significantly differently biochemically. When establishing assumptions, an approach that relates gene expression to drug targets must consider the fact that most medications bind proteins rather than DNA or RNA (Tugwell, 2011)

Making It All Clinically Relevant

Research findings will be used to enhance medical treatment for patients, as that is the ultimate goal of this study. Many of the findings from this study have not yet been used in clinical practice. It is not yet clear how to apply research findings to improve patient care, and many doctors lack the training to incorporate genetic testing for patients into their practices. Pharmacogenomics is an area where bioinformatics has the potential to have the greatest therapeutic effect.

Pharmaceutical R&D typically takes a "one size fits all" approach to solving medical problems. Drug selection, dosing, and side effects are all influenced by an individual's unique genetic make-up, and it's becoming increasingly clear that developing medications through genetic customization offers therapeutic benefits. One study revealed that the potential for adverse effects from the anticoagulant warfarin might be reduced by 60% in a hypothetical pharmacogenetically motivated clinical trial. Just two examples of medications that have been discovered to have substantial pharmacogenomic interactions are the anticoagulant clopidrogrel and the cancer therapy thiopurines.

An early example of a prospective pharmacogenomics application is a trial employing the Type II diabetes medicine rosiglitazone for Alzheimer's disease. Predictions indicated that ApoE4 non-carriers would do better than ApoE4 carriers. Preliminary Phase II pharmacogenetic data suggested that non-ApoE4 carriers fared better than placebo. Though a later analysis of patients stratified by ApoE4 found no significant advantages, the idea of prospective gene-based classification for therapy trials remains fascinating for the future. Future research requires the formulation of hypotheses on gene stratification, which calls for the development of new bioinformatics methods. New medications will lack established gene interactions; hence, tools for predicting drug-target or drug-gene interactions will be crucial.

Pharmacogenomics has already led to improvements in drug prescribing and dosing. Typically, doctors will write prescriptions with the idea that "one dosage fits all," making no considerations like patient gender, weight, liver and kidney function, or allergy history. The anticoagulant warfarin is only one example of a drug with a complicated dose formula. Until coagulation tests normalize, the dose of warfarin is generally determined using a time-consuming "guess and test" strategy. Numerous dose-modifying SNPs, such as CYP2C9 and VKORC1, have been discovered thanks to pharmacogenomics. Similar studies have been conducted on several additional medications, including clopidogrel, tramadol, antipsychotics, and many more. The International Warfarin Pharmacogenomic Consortium (IWPC) has revised its warfarin dose algorithms, and they should be available to clinicians (International Warfarin Pharmacogenetics Consortium). Doctors need to be educated and trained in personalized medicine, and more clinical research is needed to prove the efficacy of prescriptions based on pharmacogenetics.

Bioinformatics helps get research discoveries closer to the clinic by publishing them through easily accessible databases like PharmGKB, dbGaP, and PacDB. The manual curation of data presents the biggest challenge for such databases. To speed up the collection of this structured data, text mining techniques with a biological and medical focus might be used, such as those that employ natural language processing and sentence grammar to extract drug-gene and gene-gene interactions from the scientific literature. Proper planning and execution of these databases and procedures are crucial. All of these data sources are prone to inaccuracies, making data validation crucial, especially before the data is used in the clinic. Finally, the use of bioinformatics in conjunction with EMRs presents both difficulties and prospects (EMR). For instance, Vanderbilt's BioBank technology integrates anonymized electronic medical records with patient DNA to create a comprehensive resource for translational research on the linkages between genetics and health and disease. In addition to HMOs, certain other healthcare providers have also begun gathering genetic data on their patients. For the healthcare system to work with bioinformatics portals for data provision and analysis, the transition from paper to electronic medical records is essential. For clinical implementation of personalized medicine, bioinformatics will need to provide tools that enable clinicians to analyze genomic data in real-time.

What Is a Species?

The classification of species is a crucial issue in biology that has to be properly thought out and discussed. To put it another way, HUB members share our concern about how global biodiversity loss will affect local ecosystems and people's quality of life. A deeper comprehension of the fundamental mechanisms and processes that influence biodiversity, including speciation, is essential in light of the current global situation.

It is easy to establish genetic markers that distinguish species in some animals, such as mammals, where sexual reproduction is common. It is unclear if a definition of species can or should be developed or whether another concept of an "evolutionary unit," such as bacteria, would be more suitable. But to identify a species or other evolutionary unit, it is necessary to combine a wide range of data sets from many sources. The specifics include measurements on a molecular, morphological, ecological, and climatic scale. Therefore, creating methods and theories that allow the integration of vast, increasing, diverse data sets to handle species delimitation issues is a crucial component of the work. Previously, this new area of study was referred to as "integrative taxonomy." Participants concurred that "integrative taxonomy" is a significant problem in the area and that the only workable answer is to merge several data sources. It is not yet evident how to combine and order the many data kinds into a single integrated taxonomic framework.

Environmental sequencing and other methods for exploiting genomic data to define species boundaries were also hotly contested since they heavily relied on arbitrary or empirical cut-offs for sequence similarity. Applying different empirical criteria to various branches of the underlying species tree would be one enhancement that might be made. As prospective answers in this field, new statistical methods based on coalescent theory have been put forth. Furthermore, it was claimed that because data sets frequently include a mixture of sequences from inside and between species, the phylogenetic inference is now closely tied to species delimitation and population genetics methodologies. Instead, coordinated analysis and research methodologies are needed.

Data Mining

Data mining techniques are used to identify new, previously unknown, and hidden patterns in large data sets, as well as to describe and analyze such patterns in a human-readable format. Data mining approaches include clustering, classification, dependency modeling, and regression. Data mining in bioinformatics is hampered by the volume, diversity, and lack of a defined taxonomy to help in searching biological databases, as well as the heterogeneous data of different quality and provenance information they include. Another difficulty is that potential users have a broad variety of skill levels and expertise, making it difficult for database curators to establish an access mechanism that is suited for everyone. Due to the lack of biological database integration, querying many databases at once is quite difficult. As a result, it is critical to identify the important research problems in bioinformatics and to design new Data Mining approaches for scalable and efficient analysis, which necessitates the creation of new software development algorithms (Hsiao, 2012).

Software and Algorithm Development

Creating the software tools required for their extremely specialized field of inquiry is something that bioinformatics frequently wants to do. It is common to find that the algorithms used in these applications are excessively simplistic and underused. Most of the time, some type of adjustment is required to conform to the constraints and frameworks of the problems faced by other researchers. Another issue with the development of bioinformatics software tools is the construction of algorithms. Programs are computationally fairly expensive, which presents a special challenge in the field of bioinformatics; consequently, it is important to build better algorithms in terms of resource needs (Li, 2013). In the fields of sequence alignment, protein structure prediction, and protein function prediction, better approaches are desperately needed. However, practitioners in biosciences will need to develop their skills in mathematics, computers, and statistical analysis if they are to change from a mostly descriptive field to an information science. In response to the widely acknowledged skills need, universities have mostly created master's programs in bioinformatics, significantly increasing the availability of postgraduate bioinformatics education. However, it is clear that life science undergraduates need to improve their analytical and quantitative abilities (Li, 2013).

9.5. DATA TRANSLATION – TRANSLATING DATA FROM ONE FORMAT TO ANOTHER

Thanks to the advent of internet platforms that make it feasible to analyze biological data, biologists today have access to a plethora of knowledge. However, a technological barrier caused by the diversity of data forms prevents scientists from effectively utilizing the data. You'll need a lot of powerful tools to get beyond this roadblock. Grid technology may be useful for high-performance and high-throughput biological devices. Diverse biological dataset integration is a difficult and time-consuming operation.

As the integration of multiple biological data sources is essential, this necessitates the incorporation of platforms like Bio-Java into our system for data translation into XML format.

Protein Folding

The determination of protein folding speeds using amino acid sequences is one of the most urgent topics in computational and molecular biology. Biological macromolecules are present in tightly controlled states, Therefore, understanding their behavior requires acquaintance with all the conformations they inhabit. It effectively accomplishes its task by three-dimensionally forming macromolecules. Large complexes can have their structure determined; however, the initial resolution will be subpar. By examining their 3D structures, proteins have been the subject of several investigations to discover more about or calculate their folding velocities (Bowers, 2015).

Pharmacy Development and Research

Some people thought that the drug development process, from the initial laboratory findings through the human clinical trials and eventual retail distribution, may be revolutionized by bioinformatics. Structural biology and bioinformatics have supported lead optimization and target selection for lead creation by utilizing high-throughput methods of structure determination that provide powerful tools to test for fragment binding. Computer-aided drug design (CADD), a branch of pharmaceutical research, focuses on the computational modeling of drug-receptor interactions. In software, systems, and data warehouses for bioinformatics, CADD approaches are frequently utilized. Using bioinformatic tools, several intriguing drug development targets have been identified. Since inter-surface proteins are flat and similar in structure, the structural characterization and development of small molecule antagonists provide significant challenges for these systems. These issues highlight the importance of academia and business in improving bioinformatics research for medication development. Contrary to genome and proteome data, the bulk of knowledge regarding pharmaceuticals, drug metabolism, hazardous drug reactions, and bad drug effects is still accessible in print journals rather than electronic sources, which hinders the development of tools, databases, and prediction software. As more data is digitized, it is anticipated that the usage of simulation and modeling techniques to predict ADME, ADR, and toxicity will increase.

CHAPTER 10

APPLICATIONS OF BIOINFORMATICS

CONTENTS

10.1. INTRODUCTION

The scope and variety of areas where bioinformatics education and training are required are extensive. Furthermore, the training needs of the various target groups differ. For example, to be a successful bioinformatics engineer, one must be well-versed in cutting-edge algorithms, how they work, how to critically review them, and how to interpret the results. On the other hand, a bioinformatics user would need a firm understanding of the methodology and a greater emphasis on interpreting the results. The Curriculum Task Force of the ISCB Education Committee conducted research into the possibility of different user groups increasing and using fundamental bioinformatics skills. We describe the evolution of these capabilities and provide examples of their potential application to various bioinformatics education and training programs worldwide (Zhou, 2016).

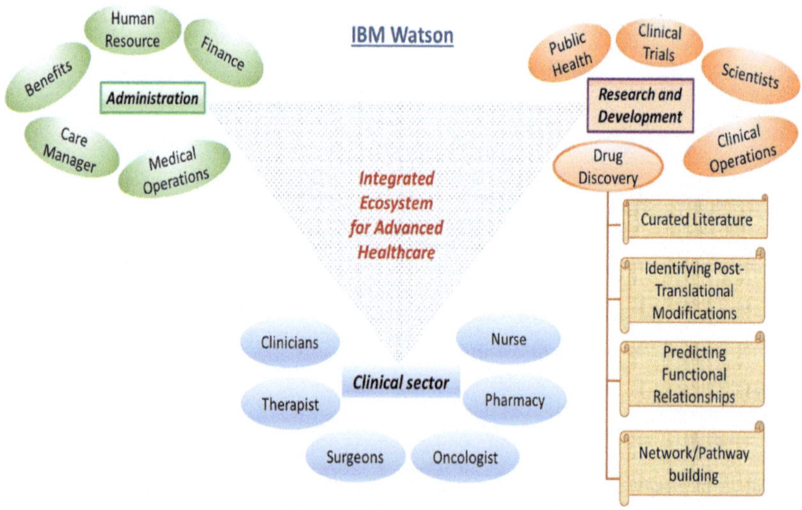

Figure 10.1: IBM Watson in healthcare data analytics.

Source: Dash, Shakyawar, Sharma, et al. Big data in healthcare: management, analysis and future prospects. J Big Data 6, 54 (2019). https://doi.org/10.1186/s40537-019-0217-0

10.2. USING BIOINFORMATICS IN AGRICULTURE

Gathering, analyzing, and interpreting genetic data are all areas in which agri-genomics, also known as agricultural genomics, is benefiting from bioinformatics breakthroughs.

The phrase "agri-informatics" refers to applying bioinformatics methodologies in agriculture for various purposes, including enhancing plant tolerance to biotic and abiotic stresses and restoring soil fertility.

Scientists have used gene discovery technologies to create focused ways to increase seed quality, provide plants with micronutrients to improve human health, and generate plants with phytoremediation capabilities (Chiusano, 2016).

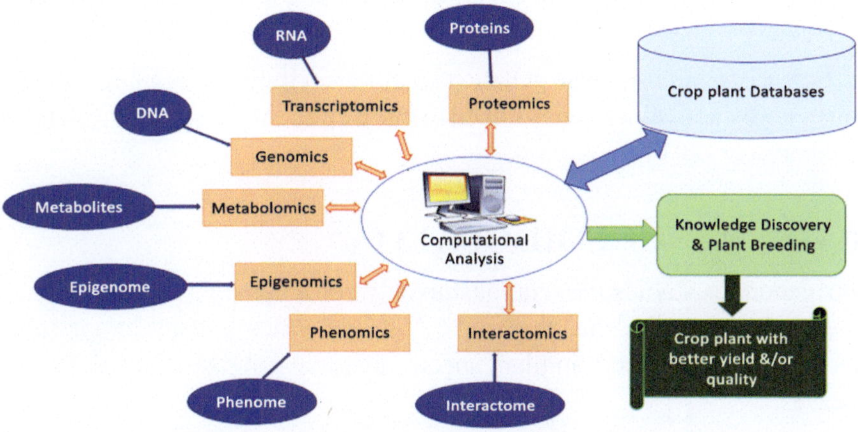

Figure 10.2: Application of bioinformatics in crop improvement,

Source: Kumar (2021). Application of Bioinformatics in Crop Improvement. In: Kumar Srivastava, D., Kumar Thakur, A., Kumar, P. (eds) Agricultural Biotechnology: Latest Research and Trends. Springer, Singapore. https://doi.org/10.1007/978-981-16-2339-4_30

Insect genomics, rather than plant genetics, is critical for understanding the processes behind biotic resistance in plants and prospective target regions. Bacillus thuringiensis, a soil-dwelling bacterium, has aroused scientists' curiosity due to the presence of proteins in its genome that are deadly to some insects.

Cotton, maize, and potato crops have had *Bacillus thuringiensis* genes put into them to improve their resistance to insect attack and minimize or eliminate the requirement for chemical treatments (Kliebenstein, 2014).

Multiple genetic manipulation methods and genomic analyses have been employed to address the issue of increasing plant tolerance to biotic and abiotic stressors. A plant's roots are especially significant regarding its capacity to withstand the detrimental impacts of abiotic stressors (Zhou,

2016). If the soil in which a plant's roots are healthy and biologically varied, it has a greater chance of surviving unfavorable conditions. Plants, despite this, are notoriously vulnerable to a wide range of climatic extremes, including drought, extreme heat, and extreme cold, and may need more time to adapt.

To protect plants from pathogens, scientists used computational and in silico genomics methods to link specific sections of DNA known as transcription factors and promoters to disease-resistant genes that encode enzymes.

Scientists can use these genetic signatures in the future to improve plant resistance by activating genes linked to more efficient resistance mechanisms (Kliebenstein, 2014).

10.3. ENHANCE SOIL QUALITY

Nutrigenomics studies the relationship between a person's genetic make-up, food preferences, and health results. Nutrigenomics is used in agriculture to look for genes in certain plant species that may give nutritional cures for diseases.

The transfer of genes to increase iron, micronutrient, and vitamin A content in rice is one agronomic application of nutrigenomics.

Because of the cognitive implications of anemia and blindness caused by iron and vitamin A deficiency, preventative therapy with increased nutritional concentrations in rice can have major ramifications.

Bioinformatics can assist researchers in increasing agricultural output and detecting dangerous chemicals in the soil. Most soils are made up of different microbial communities that are quite complicated.

Analysis of these sequences using technologies such as metagenomics sequencing revealed the presence of potentially dangerous heavy elements such as free iron and aluminum, allowing them to be excluded from future soil products (Cazorla, 2012).

10.4. EASILY ACCESSIBLE WAYS

Aside from agriculture, the economic advantage of understanding plant genomes includes disease prevention in humans and other animals. There is massive data on these biological systems, and various bioinformatics tools have been created to help with data collection, organization, and analysis.

Chloroplast DB, the Gateway of Brassica Genome, and the BGI Rice Information System are well-known plant/crop bioinformatics web databases.

10.5. THE ROLE OF BIOINFORMATICS IN MODERN PLANT BREEDING SYSTEMS

Different people have coined several phrases to define what bioinformatics is. In popular language, "bioinformatics" refers to "computer molecular biology," or the study of the molecular components of living organisms using computational methods. Applying computational, mathematical, and statistical tools to solving biological riddles by examining DNA, RNA, and amino acid sequences IS often defined as bioinformatics. According to the National Centre for Biotechnology Information, bioinformatics is the study of "the integration of biological, computational, and information technologies." Bioinformatics, which used to be primarily concerned with data management, has become inextricably linked with classical computational biology and biostatistics. This recent discovery might significantly influence biotechnology, agriculture, the environment, and possibly human health.

Bioinformatics began to take shape as a technique to accelerate biological discoveries more than ten years ago. With the publishing of the entire sequence of the *Arabidopsis thaliana* genome and the draft sequencing of the rice genome, plant science, and industry have entered the genomic era. There are several options for merging the numerous advantages of genetic data employed in systematic large-scale functional genomics initiatives (Zhou, 2016). Because of the Human Genome Project, biological knowledge has grown significantly and profoundly. Capturing, managing, processing, analyzing, and interpreting data has never been more vital. Bioinformatics is still in its infancy as a discipline of study, yet it is already showing significant promise in the developing field of biotechnology (Prasad, 2017). By providing genome information for numerous species, bioinformatics has assisted agriculture in the same way that it has aided medicine; this is especially true given the importance of bacteria in agriculture and the fact that bioinformatics gives complete genetic information for these organisms.

Plant and animal genome sequencing has aided agriculture. Plant bioinformatics seeks to encourage the release of all sequencing data into the public domain through repositories, to enable logical annotation of genes, proteins, and phenotypes, and to develop links between data on plants and data on other species, as well as data within the same species. Bioinformatics arose from the need for an appropriate informatics system to organize, administrate, and transport biological data. Still, its significance in offering tools for data analysis, interpretation, and modeling quickly became apparent. The quantity of molecular data obtained from different levels of an organism's or environmental sample's hierarchy has expanded significantly as the capabilities and affordability of omics technologies have improved. The discipline of bioinformatics has become increasingly sophisticated due to the sheer volume of data and the requirement for coordinated analysis.

Plant genomics studies the genetic and molecular origins of important physiological processes in plants that are species-specific. This knowledge is critical for generating new plant cultivars that are higher in quality and more ecologically friendly at a lower cost. The goal of this study is to present a current overview of how bioinformatics can increase breeding program efficiency and remove impediments to agricultural growth. Several branches of biology are beginning to appreciate the significance of bioinformatics. In experimental molecular biology, image and signal processing bioinformatics techniques effectively extract information from enormous volumes of raw data. It aids in identifying reported genetic and genomic alterations, as well as genome sequencing and annotation (Prasad, 2017).

Assists in the text mining of biological literature and constructing biological and gene ontologies for biological data categorization and retrieval. This discovery contributes to our understanding of how genes and proteins are regulated. Understanding evolutionary features in molecular biology necessitates comparing genetic and genomic data, which are made simpler by bioinformatics technology (Prasad, 2017). Systems biology strongly relies on finding and cataloging biological networks and pathways, which this technique promotes. Structural biology is useful for modeling and simulating molecular interactions and cellular components such as DNA, RNA, and proteins. Our program's members do research in systems biology, genomics, and proteomics. The present issue for the bioinformatics community is to provide quick and dependable access to this data and wise and inexpensive storage of the large volume of data generated.

To recover important biological data, high-tech computer approaches are required. In the pharmaceutical sector, bioinformatics technologies are rapidly employed to speed up and lower the cost of medication and molecular marker discovery and development. Perspectives on the relationship between bioinformatics and agricultural improvement. Plant breeding in the twenty-first century requires a multidisciplinary strategy for detecting and resolving breeding problems while improving agricultural productivity. In addition to state-of-the-art greenhouse equipment, genomic and bioinformatics research plays a significant role in enhancing crop yields from enhanced agricultural cultivars. However, because of the vast volumes of genotypic and phenotypic data accessible today, merging multiple data outputs for breeding is difficult. This problem will be solved, and breeding objectives will be met by incorporating phenotypes, genomes, and bioinformatics tools and resources into public and commercial breeding pipelines.

Crop breeders have traditionally depended on repeated rounds of phenotypic selection and crossing to develop superior genotypes via genetic recombination. Once genome sequences are available, all genes and genetic variations influencing agronomic qualities can be identified, and the impacts of modifications in breeding practices may be evaluated at the genotype level. Several crop breeding approaches, including genome-wide association studies and quantitative trait locus mapping, can benefit from the gene-level accuracy of agronomic variation enabled by crop population genome sequencing. For example, genomics-based breeding innovations enable the discovery of genetic variation in agricultural species, which may then be exploited to cultivate crops with exceptional climatic tolerance.

The various biological processes that compose disease resistance systems and increase crop quality may be thoroughly explored. Plant bioinformatics analyzes vast volumes of data saved in databases using specialist tools. Genomic techniques are extremely successful when it comes to complex features with a multi-genetic basis and a big environmental influence. Because of technological advancements, a small laboratory can now collect enough genetic data quickly to map quantitative trait loci in animals with no prior genomic data. As a result, genomic technologies are making it simpler to uncover QTLs and favorable, small-effect alleles previously overlooked and not incorporated into the breeding gene pool (Zhou, 2016).

REFERENCES

1. An, W., Guo, Y., Bian, Y., Ma, H., Yang, J., Li, C., & Huang, J. (2022, August). MoDNA: motif-oriented pre-training for DNA language model. In *Proceedings of the 13th ACM International Conference on Bioinformatics, Computational Biology and Health Informatics* (pp. 1-5).
2. Anderson, L. M., Petticrew, M., Rehfuess, E., Armstrong, R., Ueffing, E., Baker, P., ... & Tugwell, P. (2011). Using logic models to capture complexity in systematic reviews. *Research synthesis methods*, *2*(1), 33-42.
3. Angermueller, C., Pärnamaa, T., Parts, L., & Stegle, O. (2016). Deep learning for computational biology. *Molecular systems biology*, *12*(7), 878.
4. Aslam, B., Basit, M., Nisar, M. A., Khurshid, M., & Rasool, M. H. (2017). Proteomics: technologies and their applications. *Journal of chromatographic science*, *55*(2), 182-196.
5. Aslam, Z., Khattak, J. Z. K., Ahmed, M., & Asif, M. (2017). A role of bioinformatics in agriculture. In *Quantification of climate variability, adaptation and mitigation for agricultural sustainability* (pp. 413-434). Springer, Cham.
6. Banaganapalli, B., & Shaik, N. A. (2019). Introduction to Bioinformatics. In *Essentials of Bioinformatics, Volume I* (pp. 1-18). Springer, Cham.
7. Banerji, S., Cibulskis, K., Rangel-Escareno, C., Brown, K. K., Carter, S. L., Frederick, A. M., ... & Meyerson, M. (2012). Sequence

analysis of mutations and translocations across breast cancer subtypes. *Nature*, *486*(7403), 405-409.

8. Baslé, E., Joubert, N., & Pucheault, M. (2010). Protein chemical modification on endogenous amino acids. *Chemistry & biology*, *17*(3), 213-227.
9. Baxevanis, A. D., Bader, G. D., & Wishart, D. S. (Eds.). (2020). *Bioinformatics*. John Wiley & Sons.
10. Bonilla, N., Gutiérrez-Barranquero, J. A., de Vicente, A., & Cazorla, F. M. (2012). Enhancing soil quality and plant health through suppressive organic amendments. *Diversity*, *4*(4), 475-491.
11. Buchan, D. W., Minneci, F., Nugent, T. C., Bryson, K., & Jones, D. T. (2013). Scalable web services for the PSIPRED Protein Analysis Workbench. *Nucleic acids research*, *41*(W1), W349-W357.
12. Crist, R. C., & Berrettini, W. H. (2014). Pharmacogenetics of OPRM1. *Pharmacology Biochemistry and Behavior*, *123*, 25-33.
13. De Livera, A. M., Dias, D. A., De Souza, D., Rupasinghe, T., Pyke, J., Tull, D., ... & Speed, T. P. (2012). Normalizing and integrating metabolomics data. *Analytical chemistry*, *84*(24), 10768-10776.
14. Eaton, K. (2020). NCBImeta: efficient and comprehensive metadata retrieval from NCBI databases. *Journal of Open Source Software*, *5*(46), 1990.
15. Elias, H. G. (Ed.). (2012). *Macromolecules· 1: Volume 1: Structure and Properties*. Springer Science & Business Media.
16. Esposito, A., Colantuono, C., Ruggieri, V., & Chiusano, M. L. (2016). Bioinformatics for agriculture in the next-generation sequencing era. *Chemical and Biological Technologies in Agriculture*, *3*(1), 1-12.
17. Fokkema, I. F., Taschner, P. E., Schaafsma, G. C., Celli, J., Laros, J. F., & den Dunnen, J. T. (2011). LOVD v. 2.0: the next generation in gene variant databases. *Human mutation*, *32*(5), 557-563.
18. Forni, D., Cagliani, R., Clerici, M., & Sironi, M. (2017). Molecular evolution of human coronavirus genomes. *Trends in microbiology*, *25*(1), 35-48.
19. Gatto, L., & Christoforou, A. (2014). Using R and Bioconductor for proteomics data analysis. *Biochimica et Biophysica Acta (BBA)-Proteins and Proteomics*, *1844*(1), 42-51.
20. Gauthier, J., Vincent, A. T., Charette, S. J., & Derome, N. (2019). A

brief history of bioinformatics. *Briefings in bioinformatics*, *20*(6), 1981-1996.

21. Goujon, M., McWilliam, H., Li, W., Valentin, F., Squizzato, S., Paern, J., & Lopez, R. (2010). A new bioinformatics analysis tools framework at EMBL–EBI. *Nucleic acids research*, *38*(suppl_2), W695-W699.
22. Hartwell, L. H., Hood, L., Goldberg, M. L., Reynolds, A. E., & Silver, L. M. (2011). *Genetics: from genes to genomes*. McGraw-Hill.
23. Huang, M., Nichols, T., Huang, C., Yu, Y., Lu, Z., Knickmeyer, R. C., ... & Alzheimer's Disease Neuroimaging Initiative. (2015). FVGWAS: Fast voxelwise genome wide association analysis of large-scale imaging genetic data. *Neuroimage*, *118*, 613-627.
24. Hubbard, S. J., & Jones, A. R. (Eds.). (2010). *Proteome Bioinformatics* (Vol. 604). Totowa, NJ, USA:: Humana Press.
25. Kellis, M., Wold, B., Snyder, M. P., Bernstein, B. E., Kundaje, A., Marinov, G. K., ... & Hardison, R. C. (2014). Defining functional DNA elements in the human genome. *Proceedings of the National Academy of Sciences*, *111*(17), 6131-6138.
26. Kliebenstein, D. J. (2014). Quantitative genetics and genomics of plant resistance to insects. *Annual Plant Reviews: Insect□Plant Interactions*, *47*, 235-262.
27. Kojić-Prodić, B., & Štefanić, Z. (2010). Symmetry versus asymmetry in the molecules of life: homomeric protein assemblies. *Symmetry*, *2*(2), 884-906.
28. Kushwaha, U. K. S., Deo, I., Jaiswal, J. P., & Prasad, B. (2017). Role of bioinformatics in crop improvement. *Glob J Sci Front Res D Agric Vet*, *17*, 13-24.
29. Law, C. W., Chen, Y., Shi, W., & Smyth, G. K. (2014). voom: Precision weights unlock linear model analysis tools for RNA-seq read counts. *Genome biology*, *15*(2), 1-17.
30. Lee, D., Yang, S. M., Kim, T. H., Jeon, B. C., Kim, Y. S., Yoon, J. G., ... & Noh, T. W. (2012). Multilevel data storage memory using deterministic polarization control. *Advanced Materials*, *24*(3), 402-406.
31. Lederberg, J. (1994). The transformation of genetics by DNA: an anniversary celebration of Avery, MacLeod and McCarty (1944). *Genetics*, *136*(2), 423.
32. Li, H., & Homer, N. (2010). A survey of sequence alignment algorithms

for next-generation sequencing. *Briefings in bioinformatics, 11*(5), 473-483.

33. Liao, S. H., Chu, P. H., & Hsiao, P. Y. (2012). Data mining techniques and applications–A decade review from 2000 to 2011. *Expert systems with applications, 39*(12), 11303-11311.
34. Liu, L., Tang, L., Dong, W., Yao, S., & Zhou, W. (2016). An overview of topic modeling and its current applications in bioinformatics. *SpringerPlus, 5*(1), 1-22.
35. Low, J. T., & Weeks, K. M. (2010). SHAPE-directed RNA secondary structure prediction. *Methods, 52*(2), 150-158.
36. Madeira, F., Park, Y. M., Lee, J., Buso, N., Gur, T., Madhusoodanan, N., ... & Lopez, R. (2019). The EMBL-EBI search and sequence analysis tools APIs in 2019. *Nucleic acids research, 47*(W1), W636-W641.
37. Nissen, B., & Bowers, J. (2015, April). Data-things: digital fabrication situated within participatory data translation activities. In *Proceedings of the 33rd Annual ACM Conference on Human Factors in Computing Systems* (pp. 2467-2476).
38. Noddings, N. (2013). *Caring: A relational approach to ethics and moral education.* Univ of California Press.
39. Pabinger, S., Dander, A., Fischer, M., Snajder, R., Sperk, M., Efremova, M., ... & Trajanoski, Z. (2014). A survey of tools for variant analysis of next-generation genome sequencing data. *Briefings in bioinformatics, 15*(2), 256-278.
40. Pickett, B. E., Sadat, E. L., Zhang, Y., Noronha, J. M., Squires, R. B., Hunt, V., ... & Scheuermann, R. H. (2012). ViPR: an open bioinformatics database and analysis resource for virology research. *Nucleic acids research, 40*(D1), D593-D598.
41. Pushparaj, P. N. (2019). Journal: Essentials of Bioinformatics, Volume I, 2019, p. 287-318. *Journal: Essentials of Bioinformatics, 1*, 287-318.
42. Robinson, M. D., McCarthy, D. J., & Smyth, G. K. (2010). edgeR: a Bioconductor package for differential expression analysis of digital gene expression data. *bioinformatics, 26*(1), 139-140.
43. Shafi, A., & Zahoor, I. (2019). Bioinformatics and plant stress management. In *Essentials of Bioinformatics, Volume III* (pp. 47-78). Springer, Cham.
44. Sherry, S. T., Ward, M. H., Kholodov, M., Baker, J., Phan, L., Smigielski, E. M., & Sirotkin, K. (2001). dbSNP: the NCBI database

of genetic variation. *Nucleic acids research*, *29*(1), 308-311.

45. Singh, V. K., Singh, A. K., Chand, R., & Kushwaha, C. (2011). Role of bioinformatics in agriculture and sustainable development. *Int J Bioinforma Res*, *3*(2), 221-226.
46. Stumpfe, D., & Bajorath, J. (2011). Similarity searching. *Wiley Interdisciplinary Reviews: Computational Molecular Science*, *1*(2), 260-282.
47. Sugimoto, M., Kawakami, M., Robert, M., Soga, T., & Tomita, M. (2012). Bioinformatics tools for mass spectroscopy-based metabolomic data processing and analysis. *Current bioinformatics*, *7*(1), 96-108.
48. Tambi, R., Bayoumi, R., Lansberg, P., & Banerjee, Y. (2018). Blending gagne's instructional model with Peyton's approach to design an introductory bioinformatics lesson plan for medical students: proof-of-concept study. *JMIR Medical Education*, *4*(2), e11122.
49. Tastan Bishop, Ö., Adebiyi, E. F., Alzohairy, A. M., Everett, D., Ghedira, K., Ghouila, A., ... & H3ABioNet Consortium, as members of The H3Africa Consortium). (2015). Bioinformatics education—perspectives and challenges out of Africa. *Briefings in bioinformatics*, *16*(2), 355-364.
50. Torrisi, M., & Pollastri, G. (2019). Protein structure annotations. In *Essentials of Bioinformatics, Volume I* (pp. 201-234). Springer, Cham.
51. Welch, L., Lewitter, F., Schwartz, R., Brooksbank, C., Radivojac, P., Gaeta, B., & Schneider, M. V. (2014). Bioinformatics curriculum guidelines: toward a definition of core competencies. *PLOS computational biology*, *10*(3), e1003496.
52. Yandell, M., & Ence, D. (2012). A beginner's guide to eukaryotic genome annotation. *Nature Reviews Genetics*, *13*(5), 329-342.
53. Zahoor, I., Shafi, A., Fazili, K. M., & Haq, E. (2019). Bioinformatics and medicinal plant research: current scenario. In *Essentials of Bioinformatics, Volume III* (pp. 141-157). Springer, Cham.

INDEX

C

Q

R